COLOUR GUIDE

Accident and Emergency Medicine

David G. Ferguson MB BCh BAO FRCS(Ed)
Consultant in Accident and Emergency Medicine,
Royal Hallamshire Hospital, Sheffield, UK
Honorary Lecturer in Accident and Emergency Medicine,
University of Sheffield

David I. Fodden MB ChB FRCS(Ed) DA(UK)
Consultant in Accident and Emergency Medicine,
Pinderfields General Hospital
Wakefield, UK

JUDITH MORGAN
TEACHING AND
DEVELOPMENT SISTER

Churchill Livingstone
EDINBURGH LONDON MADRID MELBOURNE NEW YORK AND TOKYO 1993

CHURCHILL LIVINGSTONE
Medical Division of Pearson Professional Limited

Distributed in the United States of America by
Churchill Livingstone Inc., 650 Avenue of the Americas,
New York, N.Y. 10011, and by associated companies,
branches and representatives throughout the world.

© Longman Group UK Limited 1993

First published 1993
   Reprinted 1995

ISBN 0-443-04512-7

British Library Cataloguing in Publication Data
A catalogue record for this book is available from the British
Library.

Library of Congress Cataloging in Publication Data
A catalogue record for this book is available
from the Library of Congress.

Publisher
Timothy Horne

Project Editor
Jim Killgore

Production
Nancy Henry

Designer
Design Resources Unit

Sales Promotion Executive
Marion Pollock

The
publisher's
policy is to use
**paper manufactured
from sustainable forests**

Printed in Hong Kong
LYP/02

Acknowledgements

Most slide collections are built up over many years, and by swapping interesting and classical cases with colleagues. The following are those who we know have allowed us to use their own slides, but we fully acknowledge those other, unnamed colleagues from whom we have built up our collection over the years.

- Mr I G Rennie   Figures 21, 23, 24, 25 & 27.
- Mr S Ward   Figures 29 & 30.
- Mr P D Bull   Figure 38.
- Dr N A Barrington   Figures 51, 52, 60, 61 & 110.
- Mr W E G Thomas   Figure 90.
- Dr D Harris   Figure 91.
- Dr G R Kinghorn   Figures 98 & 99.
- Dr C I Harrington   Figures 135 & 188.
- Dr J K Gosnold   Figures 180, 181 & 182.
- Prof D R Triger   Figure 186.

Sheffield   D.G.F.
1993   D.I.F.

To our medical students
'You see but you do not observe.'
The memoirs of Sherlock Holmes
The Crooked Man

The creator of Sherlock Holmes, Sir Arthur Conan Doyle, was as a medical student inspired by his teacher, Mr Joseph Bell, a surgeon at the Royal Infirmary, Edinburgh, and a President of the Royal College of Surgeons of Edinburgh. Sir Arthur learned the great value of true observation which enables the clinician to glean essential general information about his patients, as well as their clinical conditions.

Sheffield   D.G.F.
1993   D.I.F.

Contents

1. The Accident and Emergency
   Department   1
2. Resuscitation   5
3. Head injuries   11
4. Eye conditions   15
5. Orofacial conditions   21
6. Ear pain   29
7. The neck   33
8. Traumatic chest pain   37
9. The shoulder   39
10. The arm   43
11. The elbow   45
12. The wrist   49
13. Hand conditions   57
14. Perianal conditions   67
15. Genitourinary problems   73
16. Hip pain   79

17. The groin   81
18. The knee   83
19. The leg   91
20. The ankle   93
21. Bursitis   97
22. Skin conditions   99
23. Soft tissue infection   105
24. Burns   111
25. Wound care   115
26. Foreign bodies   123
27. Plastering   125
28. Gunshot wounds and blast
    injuries   129
29. Non-accidental injury   131
30. Miscellaneous problems   133
31. Dangers to staff   135

Index   137

1 / The Accident and Emergency Department

The Accident and Emergency (A & E) Department is the front door of every hospital and through it will come all manner of injuries and illnesses. It is difficult to define exactly who should be seen in the unit—it could be stated that anyone with an injury more than 24 hours old should not be seen and staff often feel that patients who have self-referred have inappropriate and trivial conditions which would be better seen by their general practitioners.

The patient   The A & E Department offers an ever open door which can act as a fail-safe mechanism for the community and ensure that anyone requiring emergency treatment can always be afforded it. Remember that the public do not have the knowledge of the doctors and nurses in the A & E Department and, because of this, things which seem trivial to us may appear very serious to them.

Figure 1 shows a breakdown of patients presenting to a selection of A & E Departments. The majority of patients are 'walking wounded', and a large proportion of the stretcher cases have an acute medical disorder. Between 20 and 25% of patients fall into the paediatric age group.

The team   The A & E Department has a large team (Fig. 2) of staff who work closely with the community through general practitioners and the ambulance service. Within the department, because of the nature of the work and, in particular, because of the emergency and stressful situations that can arise, it is essential that everyone works as a team. Domestics, porters, ECG technicians, social workers, secretaries, reception staff, doctors and nurses, all form part of the team and no one individual is more important than another.

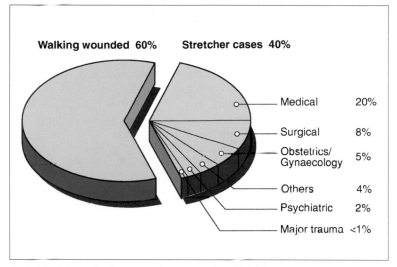

Fig. 1 A breakdown of patients presenting to a selection of A & E Departments.

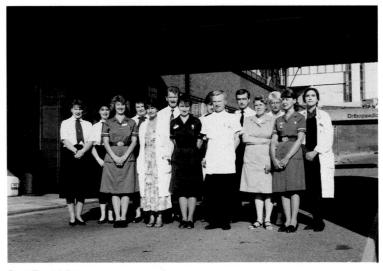

Fig. 2 The A & E team.

The workload of an A & E department can broadly be divided into major (trolley) cases and minor (walking wounded) cases.

Major cases Those conditions presenting to the trolley area may require resuscitation, and generally consist of serious medical and surgical conditions (Fig. 3). Major trauma is not common and the majority of the workload consists of acute medical emergencies. With the improved medical and social care in the community, there are more elderly cases coming to hospital and the average age of those being seen is now greater than that a few years ago. This creates bed management problems as the elderly often require prolonged rehabilitation.

Minor cases The area catering for walking wounded deals with sprains, strains, minor fractures and wounds (Fig. 4). The biggest problem with this work is that it tends to be very repetitive and there is a great temptation to be less careful when examining and documenting such cases. The majority of litigation against A & E departments stems from such errors.

There is a wealth of pathology in this area, if the staff are astute enough to note it, even though it may not be related directly to the presenting complaint. This is an excellent area to learn to work quickly and efficiently.

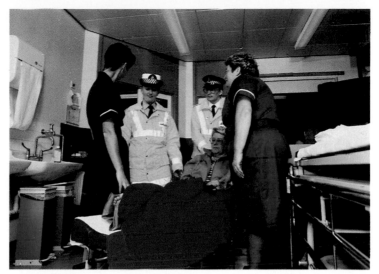

Fig. 3 Reception of a patient on the majors area.

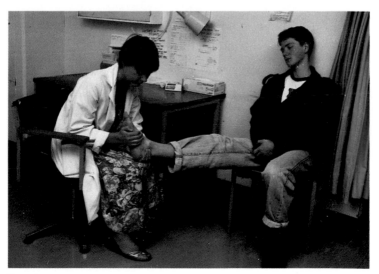

Fig. 4 A case in the minors area.

2 / Resuscitation

General points   The management of a cardiorespiratory arrest is
something which demands smooth, efficient teamwork
(Fig. 5) between medical, nursing and paramedical staff
if a successful outcome is to be achieved. Frequent
rehearsal using manikins and critical self-audit are
necessary as are adequate numbers of staff. Each team
member should have a clearly defined role (Fig. 6) and
one should be elected as team leader. All major decisions
should be directed through this person and he/she
should not take any active role in the resuscitation.
The Resuscitation Council of the United Kingdom
has produced, now well established, guidelines for the
management of this condition and all medical and
nursing personnel must be fully familiar with these.

The relatives   In the event of an unsuccessful resuscitation, it is
important to consider the relatives. They should be
told in simple words what has happened and of what
resuscitative efforts were made. It is usual practice in
England for the Coroner to be informed of all A & E
deaths and this should be explained as a routine
procedure to the relatives. Although a post-mortem
examination may be ordered, it is not uncommon for the
general practitioner to be willing to sign the death
certificate if he has seen the patient recently and is happy
that the cause of death was likely to have been due to
some serious previously diagnosed condition, such as
ischaemic heart disease.

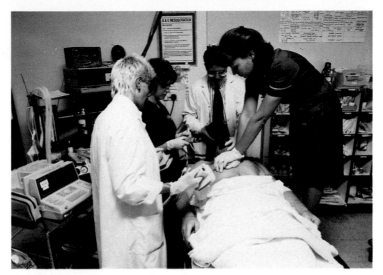

Fig. 5 The resuscitation team at work.

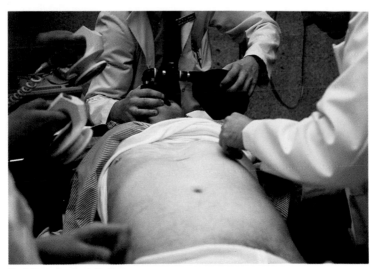

Fig. 6 Preparing for defibrillation.

Careful attention to detail is important and should be paid in every case.

Cardiac massage

Standard external cardiac massage should be undertaken with the heel of the hand on the lower part of the sternum. The depth of compression is between 3 and 5 centimetres at a rate of approximately 80 per minute. The operator should change when fatigue develops lest the technique varies and mediastinal contusions or chest wall fractures occur (Fig. 7).

Ventricular fibrillation

The standard electrode positions (Fig. 8) are just to the right of the sternum below the clavicle and at the apex. However, in refractory ventricular fibrillation, it may be necessary to defibrillate in the anteroposterior direction with the patient on their side. Alternatively, it may be necessary to change the paddles or the defibrillator in case the machine or paddles are faulty.

The paddles must not make direct contact with the skin as this will result in burning due to the high skin resistance (Fig. 9). Gel pads reduce the resistance between the paddles and the skin. They must be fresh and not placed over ECG monitor leads.

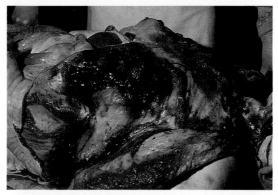

Fig. 7 Bruising and fractured ribs at post-mortem after prolonged resuscitation.

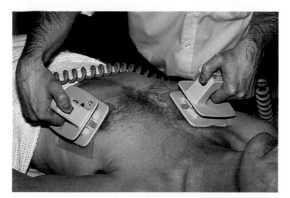

Fig. 8 The correct position for the defibrillator paddles.

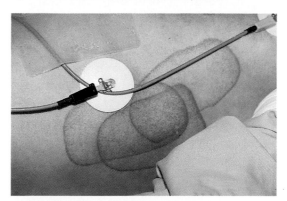

Fig. 9 Defibrillator burns resulting from poor technique.

Electro-
mechanical
dissociation

The two most easily identified causes are a tension pneumothorax and cardiac tamponade.

Tension pneumothorax. This is diagnosed by inserting a hypodermic needle through the 2nd intercostal space in the mid-clavicular line. If the needle is attached to a syringe full of saline, escaping air is detected easily on aspiration (Fig. 10). The needle can be replaced by a large bore cannula allowing time for the insertion of a chest drain.

Cardiac tamponade. A tamponade is diagnosed and treated by aspiration. A long, wide bore needle is inserted just to the left of the xiphoid cartilage and aimed upwards and backwards towards the left shoulder at 45° to the skin (Fig. 11). A monitor lead attached to the needle shows an altered pattern of electrical activity when it touches the epicardium.

Central venous
cannulation

Central venous cannulation is an elective procedure. A high approach (Fig. 12) to the internal jugular vein is the preferable route since this carries the least risk of producing a pneumothorax. The patient is put in a 15° head down position to distend the veins and minimize the risk of air embolism. The head is turned to the opposite side and the needle inserted through the skin at the level of the thyroid cartilage, just lateral to the carotid artery. It is aimed 30° to 45° backwards and towards the ipsilateral nipple. Successful puncture is made at a depth of between 2 and 7 centimetres.

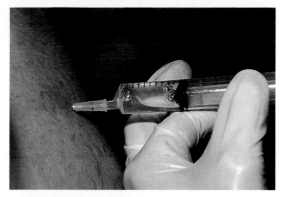

Fig. 10 Bubbles in the syringe confirm the diagnosis of a pneumothorax.

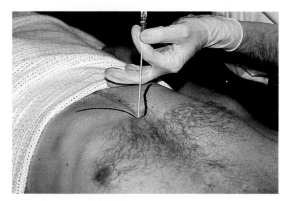

Fig. 11 Tapping a cardiac tamponade.

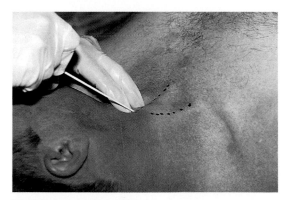

Fig. 12 Central venous cannulation.

3 / Head injuries

Presentation

Head injuries are common and often present to an A & E department following a road traffic accident or a fight. In these situations, alcohol may play a large part in the patient's clinical state. The smell of alcohol is no indication of the volume which might have been consumed. Alcohol may confuse the issue because there are common features between alcohol excess and a head injury such as loss of consciousness, confusion and aggression. Always assume that these are the result of the head injury rather than alcohol. If in doubt, admit the patient for observation.

Level of consciousness

Loss of consciousness following trauma may result from a head injury or hypovolaemia and hypoxia. These must be corrected and the patient's neurological state reassessed, as well as treating other concurrent injuries.

Scalp wounds

These are initially difficult to assess (Fig. 13) due to blood in the hair. When the wound has been cleaned, it may look less severe than was originally thought (Fig. 14). Feel gently with a gloved finger in the wound to detect any underlying fracture (Fig. 15). Scalp wounds may bleed heavily but they are not a cause of hypovolaemia in adults—if present, look for another cause.

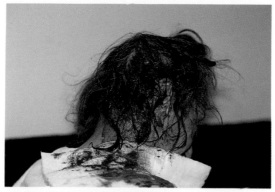

Fig. 13 Scalp laceration on arrival.

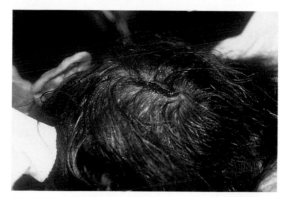

Fig. 14 Scalp laceration after cleaning.

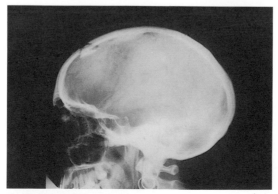

Fig. 15 Depressed skull fracture.

Skull fractures

Clinical signs

An increase of the intracranial pressure may cause compression of the oculomotor nerve against the tentorium cerebelli and produce ipsilateral dilatation of the pupil. It is important to exclude other causes of unequal pupils such as direct trauma to the eye, the application of medication (Fig. 16) or a glass eye.

Anterior cranial fossa fractures: can cause cerebrospinal fluid (CSF) rhinorrhoea, marked periorbital haematomata (panda eyes), associated with subconjunctival haemorrhage (Fig. 17). Bloody CSF rhinorrhoea may be identified by dropping some of the fluid on to blotting paper—if CSF is present, there will be a central ring of blood with a peripheral halo of CSF.

Middle cranial fossa fractures: produce a haemotympanum and, if the membrane is ruptured, blood and CSF leakage from the ear (Fig. 18). Posterior auricular bruising may also occur (Battle's sign)—usually later.

Investigations

It is more important to observe the patient's level of consciousness than to the take X-rays of the skull. Skull X-rays are notoriously difficult to interpret, particularly if the patient is restless and the quality of the film is suboptimal. Computerized tomography is the examination of choice to diagnose intracranial haemorrhage.

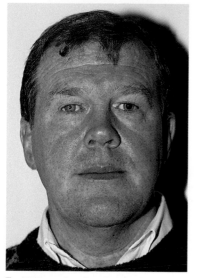

Fig. 16 Unequal pupils—dilated with cyclopentolate.

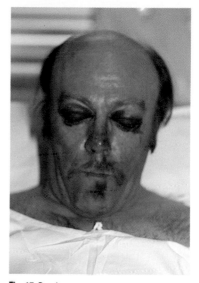

Fig. 17 Panda eyes.

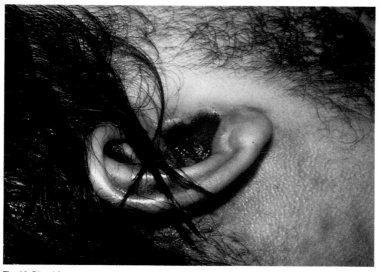

Fig. 18 Blood from ear.

4 / Eye conditions

Trauma

Aetiology   A direct blow to the eye may damage the eyelids, globe or bony wall of the orbit and, of these, the floor is the most often injured.

Clinical features   **Fracture**. A fracture produces a periorbital haematoma, local tenderness, a palpable step and a subconjunctival haemorrhage. If the posterior limit of the haemorrhage is not visible, assume that there is a fracture. There may be altered sensation in the distribution of the infraorbital nerve. A fracture which involves the floor of the orbit but not the free margin is a blow-out fracture. This, in addition to the features described above, produces enophthalmos and trapping of the infraorbital structures (Fig. 19). X-rays confirm the fracture and there is opacity of the maxillary sinus (Fig. 20). Tomography or a CT scan may be required to delineate the blow-out fracture.

Hyphaemia. A hyphaema is a collection of blood in the anterior chamber, resulting from damage to vessels on the iris (Fig. 21).

Treatment   The patient is advised not to blow the nose and prophylactic antibiotics are usually prescribed. Displaced zygomatic fractures require surgical correction as do those blow-out fractures which trap the infraorbital structures.

A patient suffering from a hyphaema should be referred to an ophthalmologist. If the patient does not rest, there is a risk of further bleeding and this is associated with a rise of the intraocular pressure which may require specific treatment.

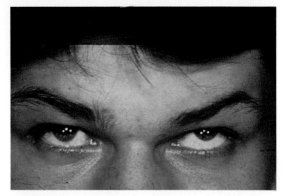

Fig. 19 Limitation of upward gaze resulting from a blow-out fracture.

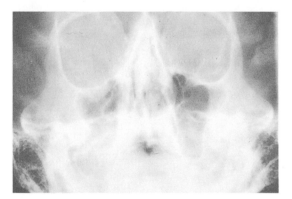

Fig. 20 'Tear drop' soft tissue swelling at the roof of the maxillary antrum.

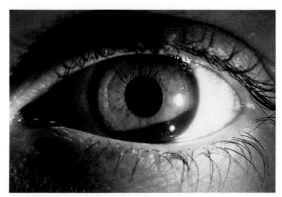

Fig. 21 A hyphaema.

Pain

Aetiology

Pain may result from surface structures or deeper structures. Surface pain results from conjunctival or scleral irritation. This may be due to a foreign body, primary conjunctivitis (Fig. 22), a corneal abrasion, scleritis or episcleritis.

Clinical features

The visual acuity should be assessed in both eyes using normal visual aids. It is usually normal. There may be photophobia, epiphora, conjunctival redness and blepharospasm. The whole of the anterior surface of the globe must be examined carefully and the eyelids everted (Fig. 23). Given a history of a high velocity fragment, X-rays must be taken of the orbital contents to exclude an intraocular foreign body even if one is seen on the surface. Staining of the cornea with fluorescein shows any corneal epithelial defect.

Treatment

Metallic corneal foreign bodies. When seen within the first few hours, these may be removed easily under local anaesthesia but, if present for longer, there may be an associated 'rust-ring' (Fig. 24). This is difficult to remove in its entirety and it is preferable to apply a firm eye-pad, give a topical antibiotic and refer to an ophthalmologist at 72 hours for its removal.

Conjunctivitis. This condition is treated with topical antibiotics for 72 hours and a firm eye-pad.

Scleritis and episcleritis. These are occasionally associated with systemic disorders such as rheumatoid disease and inflammatory bowel disease, and the eye condition is best treated by an ophthalmologist.

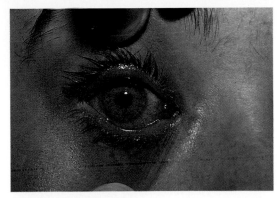

Fig. 22 Bacterial conjunctivitis.

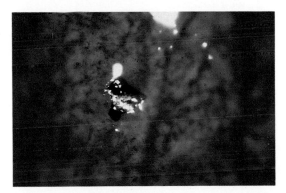

Fig. 23 Metallic foreign body beneath the upper eyelid.

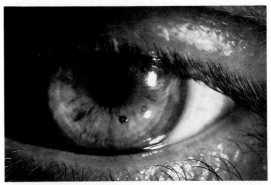

Fig. 24 Rust-ring at 48 hours after removal of a foreign body.

Other important causes of pain

These include the following:
- a dendritic ulcer
- acute glaucoma
- acute iritis
- perforating injury.

Clinical features **Dendritic ulcer**: a corneal ulcer of viral aetiology. It causes symptoms of conjunctivitis but does not respond to antibiotics. Fluorescein staining reveals the typical branched ulcer (Fig. 25). Topical steroids are absolutely contraindicated.

Acute glaucoma: a condition associated with pain in the eye and diminished visual acuity. The globe is palpably firm, the cornea hazy and the pupil oval and non-reactive to light. It may arise de novo or be secondary to anticholinergic drugs.

Iritis: inflammation of the anterior uveal tract which causes intense pain and photophobia. The pupil is small and the redness is initially around the cornea (Fig. 26). The consensual light reflex causes pain in the affected eye.

Perforating injury: should be suspected with a history of a high velocity missile, e.g. metal striking metal. There may be a scleral or corneal wound which may not be obvious. The iris may prolapse through a corneal wound producing a tear-shaped pupil (Fig. 27).

Treatment Early referral to an ophthalmologist should be made in all of these cases since serious complications can develop or the systemic disease which precipitated the condition requires investigation and treatment.

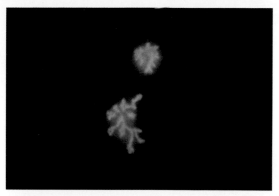

Fig. 25 Fluorescein-stained dendritic ulcer under ultraviolet light.

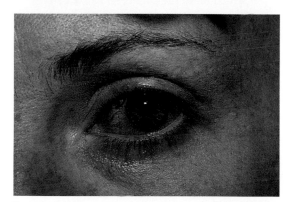

Fig. 26 Acute iritis.

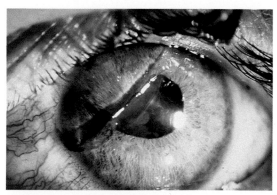

Fig. 27 Iris prolapse through a corneal wound.

5 / Orofacial conditions

Dental problems

Trauma

Subluxation or dislocation of a tooth results from trauma. If a tooth has been dislocated, it can be stored in milk or in the buccal sulcus pending relocation.

Treatment   The tooth should be cleaned carefully and replaced in its socket as soon as possible, then splinted. The longer the delay in reducing a subluxed or dislocated tooth, the greater is the chance of damage to the neurovascular structures in the pulp (Fig. 28). If a tooth has been dislocated and cannot be found, X-ray the chest to ensure that it has not been inhaled. The usual site at which it will lodge is in the right main bronchus (Fig. 29).

The bleeding socket

Treatment   This is treated by rolling a gauze swab and placing it directly across the socket. The patient is advised to bite firmly for 15 minutes. If unsuccessful (Fig. 30), a horizontal mattress suture may be placed across the neck of the socket. It does not close the socket but tightens the gingiva, so arresting mucosal bleeding. If this fails, a plug of a haemostatic material should be inserted into the socket prior to suture.

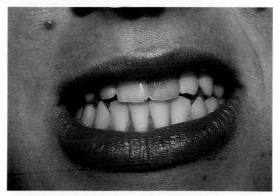

Fig. 28 Discolouration of a dislocated tooth resulting from damage to the pulp.

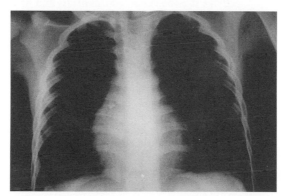

Fig. 29 Inhaled tooth in the right main bronchus.

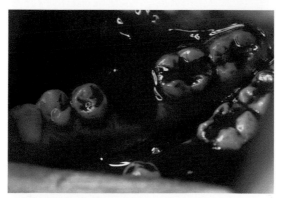

Fig. 30 A bleeding tooth socket.

Nasal problems

Trauma
This may result in deformity and marked swelling.

Treatment There is no need to X-ray the nose unless a compound fracture is suspected. The nasal bridge is tender and deviated (Fig. 32) and this is best seen from above. The patency of the nasal airways should be checked and a septal haematoma (Fig. 31) looked for. This looks like a cherry in the middle of the nose and, if present, immediate ENT referral should be made since the septal cartilage may be rendered ischaemic and will perforate, particularly if an abscess develops. A patient with a suspected nasal fracture is usually referred to an ENT surgeon at between 5 and 10 days from the date of the injury to decide if reduction is necessary.

Epistaxis
This occurs usually at the extremes of life and may result from trauma, mucosal inflammation or spontaneous haemorrhage (Fig. 33) from atherosclerotic vessels associated occasionally with hypertension. The septum may bleed anteriorly from Little's area or from more posteriorly.

Treatment
- *Anterior bleeding* may be controlled readily by pinching the nose firmly, but occasionally it is necessary to cauterize the vessel or pack the nose.
- *Posterior bleeding* should be treated by an ENT surgeon since this usually requires packing and may necessitate early surgery.

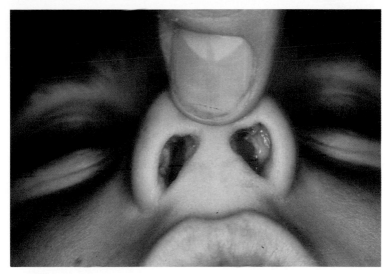

Fig. 31 Septal haematoma.

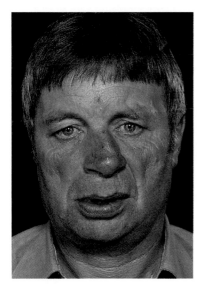

Fig. 32 Frontal view of a deviated nasal bridge.

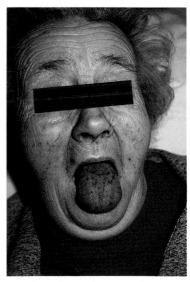

Fig. 33 Hereditary haemorrhagic telangiectasia resulting in epistaxis.

Lip injuries

Full thickness wounds are common and are due to direct trauma from outside or a tooth biting through the lip.

Treatment The wound edges should be debrided and then closed in layers to avoid the development of a salivary fistula. A wound through the vermilion border (Fig. 34) must be repaired very carefully since the slightest irregularity of the scar leaves a cosmetically obvious appearance.

Mucosal lacerations heal very well. They initially become macerated and ulcerated and the patient should be advised to use a saline or antiseptic mouthwash and take care with dental hygiene.

Jaw injuries

Dislocation

Dislocation usually occurs without trauma. Typically, the patient yawns, feels pain in front of the ear and is unable to close the mouth properly (Fig. 35).

Treatment X-rays confirm the dislocation and reduction is effected easily by firm downward and backward pressure on the lower molar teeth.

Fracture

A fracture of the mandible is not always obvious clinically. Palpate carefully the whole of the mandible and look for misalignment of the teeth, swelling, bleeding or sub-lingual bruising which, if present, is pathognomonic of the diagnosis until proven otherwise. X-ray the mandible and be careful to maintain the patient's airway, particularly if the level of consciousness is depressed.

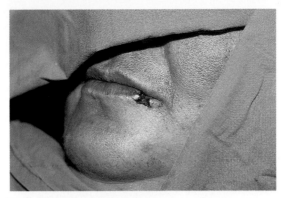

Fig. 34 Wound at the vermilion border.

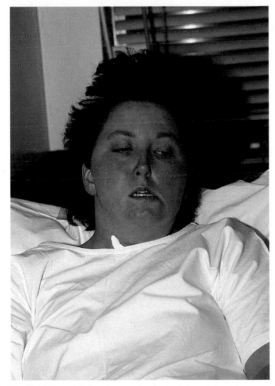

Fig. 35 Unilateral dislocation causing in deviation of the chin.

Throat problems

Clinical features Patients often present complaining of having swallowed something which has lodged in the throat. The position of the foreign body is not well localized and there is dysphagia. Rarely there may be dyspnoea and dysphonia and, if the foreign body has perforated the airway, there will be surgical emphysema.

Examination Inspect the mouth carefully, the tonsillar area (Fig. 36) and the posterior third of the tongue, behind the vallate papillae. It is possible to examine the larynx indirectly with a mirror but this takes practice and the patient's confidence must be gained. X-rays of the soft tissues of the neck may visualize a foreign body (Fig. 37) and show any associated surgical emphysema. However, foreign bodies are often difficult to identify, particularly in a patient with heavily calcified laryngeal cartilages.

Treatment If the foreign body is identified in the oropharynx, remove it. It may be necessary to spray the oropharynx with topical local anaesthetic and, if this is done, warn the patient not to eat or drink until the sensation has returned to normal. When the foreign body has been removed, warn the patient to expect the abnormal sensation to persist for several days until the mucosal wound has healed.

If the foreign body is not visible and the patient has significant symptoms such as drooling of saliva, dysphagia or dyspnoea, ask for an urgent ENT opinion.

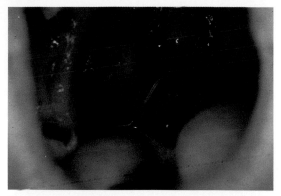

Fig. 36 Fish bone lodged in the right tonsillar area.

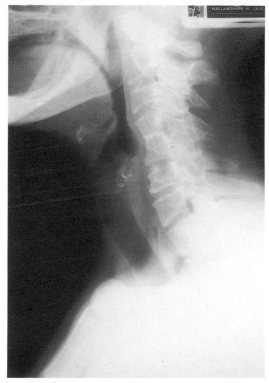

Fig. 37 Glass foreign body in the oesophagus at the C7/T1 level.

6 / **Ear pain**

Inflammatory conditions

Aetiology   ***Otitis externa***: occurs commonly in those engaged in water sports. The inflammation may be allergic, bacterial or fungal in origin (Fig. 38).

Otitis media: occurs most commonly in children as part of an upper respiratory tract infection.

Clinical features   ***Otitis externa***: causes itching of the external ear canal, a watery discharge and conductive deafness.

Otitis media: causes severe throbbing pain, fever and conductive deafness.

Examination   There is tenderness of the tragus and movements of the jaw are painful. There may be excoriation of the skin and the external ear canal is oedematous.

Otitis media is associated with redness and bulging of the ear-drum.

Treatment   ***Otitis externa***: local cleansing along with instillation of combined steroid and antibiotic drops or cream. Alternatively, a wick soaked in this preparation may be inserted and changed after 24 hours. The condition may be slow to resolve.

Otitis media: systemic antibiotics. If treated inadequately, otitis media with an effusion may develop in children. If there is frank pus behind the ear-drum, it should be drained surgically by an ENT surgeon.

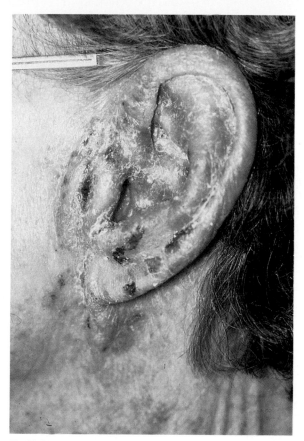

Fig. 38 Otitis externa.

Non-infective conditions

Aetiology
- A perichondral haematoma (Fig. 39) is caused by direct trauma to the external ear.
- Wounds through the cartilage of the ear are traumatic in origin (Fig. 41).
- Traumatic perforation of the ear-drum is due to a direct injury, e.g. scratching the ear canal with a pointed object, or by a high pressure air wave as a result of a blow to the side of the head.
- Foreign bodies may be in the meatus or embedded in the pinna (Fig. 40).

Clinical features
The perichondrium is stripped away from the cartilage and there is a boggy, tender swelling.

Perforation of the ear-drum leads to conductive deafness and a bloody discharge.

Treatment
The haematoma should be aspirated under sterile conditions and a firm dressing applied to the contours of the ear. Alternatively, a small suction drain may be introduced via the posterior surface of the ear to drain the haematoma and minimize the chance of its recurrence. This is an ENT procedure.

When an extensive injury damages skin and cartilage, the cartilaginous skeleton should be reconstructed carefully. The irregular skin edges should be trimmed to allow accurate closure to obtain a cosmetically acceptable result.

Meatal foreign bodies are often small round objects and are best removed under general anaesthetic but those in the pinna can usually be removed under local anaesthetic from the back of the pinna.

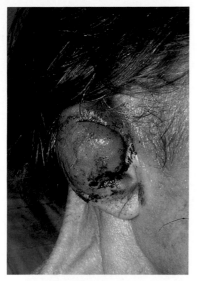

Fig. 39 A perichondral haematoma.

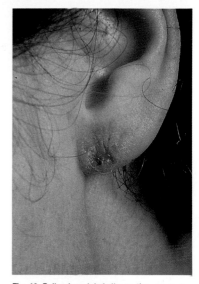

Fig. 40 Following nickel allergy, the ear stud has become embedded in the pinna.

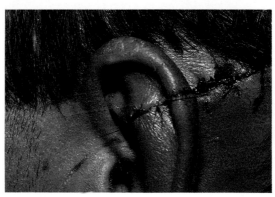

Fig. 41 A sutured machete wound to the ear.

7 / The neck

Pain

Aetiology

Sprain. A sprain of the cervical spine occurs most commonly in a rear impact road traffic accident. It causes hyperextension of the cervical spine followed rapidly by flexion (whiplash injury).

Torticollis. Spontaneous onset of pain in the neck may be due to acute torticollis (Fig. 42). This is due to spasm in the large muscles of the neck. It is of unknown aetiology.

Clinical features

Sprain. There may be transient neurological symptoms and the neck is usually pain free initially. Pain and stiffness develop gradually and X-rays show a straight cervical spine which is evidence of spasm.

Torticollis. This occurs in young adults and is associated with the neck held flexed and the head rotated to one side. There are no abnormal neurological signs.

Treatment

Sprain. There are several methods which include immobilization in a firm or soft cervical collar (Figs 43 & 44) until the patient is pain free. There is a trend towards early mobilization with or without active physiotherapy. The acute symptoms of a whiplash injury may last up to 8 weeks but a less intense discomfort may develop and this may last for months.

Torticollis. This resolves quickly and medication with painkillers and muscle relaxants (such as diazepam) resolve the symptoms within a few days.

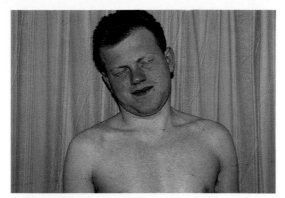

Fig. 42 Torticollis.

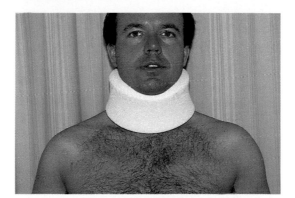

Fig. 43 Anterior view of a soft cervical collar.

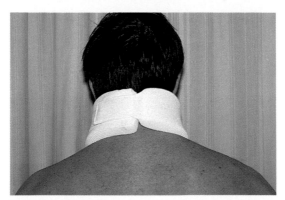

Fig. 44 Posterior view of a soft cervical collar showing the Velcro fastener.

Wounds

Aetiology   They may be self-inflicted (Fig. 45) or due to an assault
(Fig. 46). In either case, the motive is death. Occasionally
a wound may result from an accident.

Clinical features   The self-inflicted wound usually has 'intention' marks.
These are short, superficial wounds which increase in
depth and length until the major wound is produced.
Wounds resulting from an assault are usually single and
deep.

Treatment   Cover with a moist dressing and apply direct pressure.
The patient can sit up and this will decrease
haemorrhage; however, this position increases the risk of
air embolism. If the patient is hypotensive, or there are
other injuries present, it may be necessary to lie him
down but this will tend to increase the haemorrhage.
Other injuries must be sought and treated. Clamping
vessels blindly must not be attempted.

Wounds which penetrate the platysma should be
explored formally in theatre but more superficial wounds
may be sutured in the department after careful
inspection.

Damage to the upper airway should be assessed
carefully and an experienced anaesthetist and ENT
surgeon consulted early.

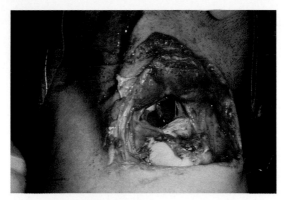

Fig. 45 Self-inflicted throat laceration.

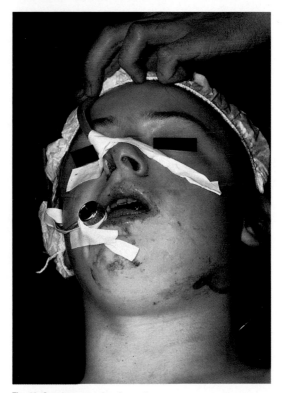

Fig. 46 Gunshot wound to the neck.

8 / Traumatic chest pain

Non-penetrating injuries

Aetiology
- *Direct injuries* occur most commonly as a result of a fall, sport or an assault.
- *Indirect injuries* occur in pathologically weakened bone such as in postmenopausal women, patients on steroids or those with disseminated malignancy.

Clinical features
There is marked tenderness over the area of the injury. A deceleration injury resulting from a road traffic accident produces characteristic bruising (Fig. 47) and an ECG may show evidence of myocardial injury.

The diagnosis of a rib fracture does not require an X-ray but an X-ray is required if there is suspicion of associated pathology such as a chest infection or a pneumothorax.

Treatment
Strapping the ribs around half the circumference of the chest wall (Fig. 48) gives good pain relief and does not limit respiration, providing that an elasticated strapping is used. Analgesia must be provided and this may be systemic or by a regional nerve block. Advice regarding breathing exercises should be given to minimize the likelihood of a chest infection developing.

Penetrating injuries

These are uncommon and are due to assault (Fig. 49) or accident. The major life-threatening conditions of a tension pneumothorax or cardiac tamponade must be sought and treated immediately. Penetrating cardiac injuries must be treated by immediate thoracotomy and closure of the myocardial defect.

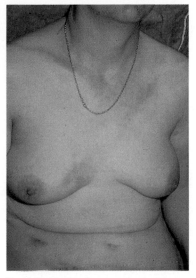

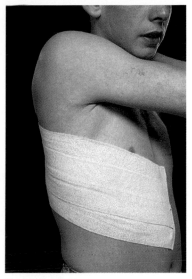

Fig. 47 Seat belt marks across the chest and abdomen.

Fig. 48 Rib strapping.

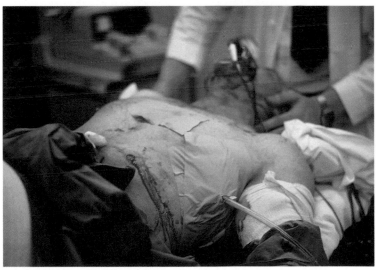

Fig. 49 Stabbing to the chest and abdomen.

9 / The shoulder

Anatomy Stability of the glenohumeral joint is sacrificed in favour of the large range of movement which is permitted. The bony contours and labrum glenoidale contribute little to stability, this being afforded primarily by the tendons of the rotator cuff and the ligaments.

Anterior dislocation

This occurs typically in young adults and results from a fall on to the outstretched hand.

Clinical features There is pain, spasm and the rounded contour of the deltoid is replaced by the square contour of the acromion (Fig. 50). Neuropraxia of the brachial plexus or axillary nerve occurs infrequently but should be sought prior to reduction.

Treatment There are several methods of reduction, including the Hippocratic, Kocher, Stimson and Milch manoeuvres. The technique used should be dictated by local policy. Entonox may suffice as the method of analgesia but an opiate is usually required in addition. General or regional anaesthesia may be needed in more muscular patients.

Posterior dislocation

This occurs much less frequently and is seen particularly in epileptics or those having suffered an electric shock.

Clinical features The contour of the shoulder is normal. The X-ray reveals the 'light-bulb' deformity (symmetry of the humeral head) and it stands off more than usual from the glenoid (Fig. 51). An axial view is essential to confirm the diagnosis (Fig. 52).

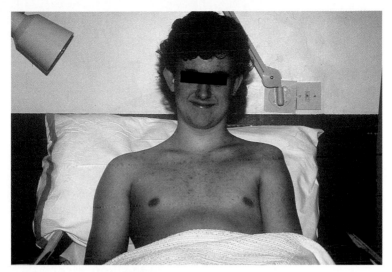

Fig. 50 Anterior dislocation of the left shoulder.

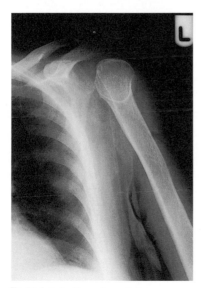

Fig. 51 Anterior X-ray of a posterior dislocation of the left shoulder.

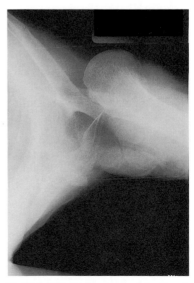

Fig. 52 Axial X-ray of a posterior dislocation of the left shoulder.

Painful arc

This is pain arising from the shoulder itself or the associated soft tissues and is felt typically in the middle one third of abduction (Fig. 53).

Aetiology
- Calcific bursitis (Fig. 54)
- Degenerative rotator cuff disease
- Degenerative disease of the acromioclavicular joint

Clinical features The pain may be of spontaneous onset, radiates to the insertion of the deltoid muscle and is of an aching nature. There may be limitation of rotation at the shoulder joint.

Treatment This is directed at reducing local inflammation using physiotherapy, non-steroidal anti-inflammatory agents and maintaining mobility by gentle exercises. Local steroid injections may be of benefit but strict asepsis must be observed.

Acromioclavicular injuries

Acromioclavicular separation may be divided into 1st, 2nd and 3rd degree, depending upon the amount of separation seen radiographically.

Aetiology A fall on to the point of the shoulder, usually in young sportsmen.

Clinical features Local tenderness and deformity (Fig. 55). There is painful limitation of movement and X-rays exclude a fracture of the outer end of the clavicle.

Treatment Analgesia and a triangular bandage followed by gentle exercises produce good results although the deformity generally persists.

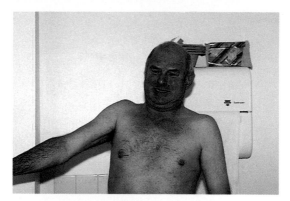

Fig. 53 Painful limitation of abduction.

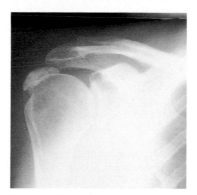

Fig. 54 Calcification in the subacromial bursa.

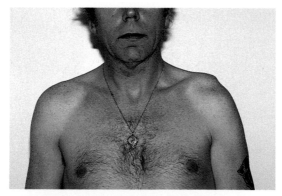

Fig. 55 Complete separation of the left acromioclavicular joint.

10 / The arm

Damage to the biceps muscle

Aetiology
The long head of the biceps muscle is thought to rupture due to avascular degeneration and thus is a condition of the over 50s. The distal attachment may rupture due to similar pathology or due to scarring from previous injury. A direct blow to the biceps may result from an assault or contact sport and cause an intramuscular haematoma.

Clinical features
The patient will generally have been stressing his arm when he feels something go. If the injury has occurred recently, there will be pain on contracting the biceps. The free head contracts up or down the arm and appears as a swelling over its anterior aspect (Fig. 56). After a few days, heavy bruising may develop down the arm (Fig. 57).

Treatment
Rupture of the long head is treated conservatively using analgesia, a broad arm sling and then mobilization. Distal rupture is usually treated operatively because of the weakness of elbow flexion produced by damage to the tendon.

Direct damage to the biceps muscle may result in myositis ossificans and subsequent fibrosis within the muscle belly (Fig. 58). Such scarring is likely to be stimulated by early, vigorous mobilization so this must be avoided.

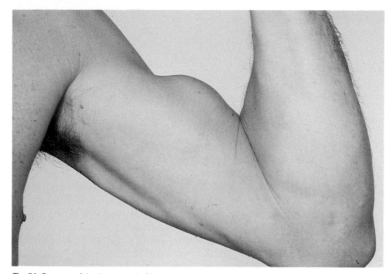

Fig. 56 Rupture of the long head of the biceps.

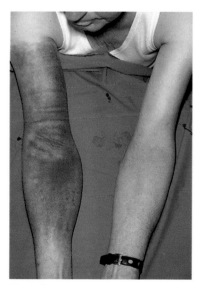

Fig. 57 Heavy bruising resulting from an acute rupture of the biceps tendon.

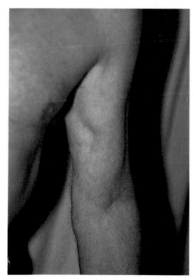

Fig. 58 Scarring of the muscle belly resulting from a previous direct injury.

11 / The elbow

Trauma

Aetiology   The usual mechanism is a fall on to the outstretched hand although direct trauma may also result in bony or ligamentous damage.

Clinical features   There may be swelling and deformity at the elbow (Fig. 59). The olecranon and epicondyles normally form an equilateral triangle—dislocation disrupts this relationship whilst a supracondylar fracture maintains it. A fracture of the olecranon produces marked local swelling, bruising and the bony prominence may not be palpable. There may be abnormal movement with crepitus around the joint and it is particularly important to check the distal neurovascular function since urgent reduction must be effected if there is any compromise.

X-ray   This demonstrates the bony injury but care must be taken in children to check the epiphyseal centres (Fig. 60) which can be displaced minimally but cause significant functional deficit subsequently. If there is no obvious bone or joint injury, check for the presence of an effusion. This raises the intracapsular but extrasynovial fat pads which appear as dark sail-like shadows anterior and posterior to the distal humerus (Fig. 61).

Treatment   A displaced injury must be reduced urgently. Displaced epicondylar or olecranon fractures are fixed internally whilst displaced radial head fractures are either excised or fixed, according to local policy. Non-displaced fractures of the radial head are treated conservatively.

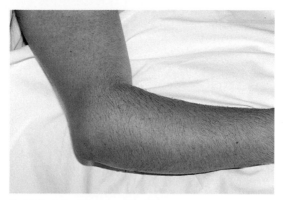

Fig. 59 Posterior dislocation of the elbow.

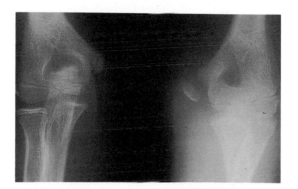

Fig. 60 Separation of the medial epicondylar epiphysis.

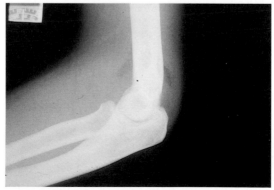

Fig. 61 Anterior and posterior fat pads.

Tendinitis

Aetiology   Epicondylitis and biceps tendinitis are due to unaccustomed repetitive activity. Epicondylitis is rarely due to playing tennis or golf.

Clinical features   There is pain and tenderness over the tendon attachment. Resisted movements of the wrist produce pain at the elbow in the case of epicondylitis (Fig. 62). Biceps tendinitis is associated with pain caused by resisted flexion of the elbow (Fig. 63) or resisted supination of the forearm.

Treatment   The elbow should be rested and a course of non-steroidal anti-inflammatory drugs should be given. If the symptoms fail to resolve, an injection of steroid and local anaesthetic around the point of maximum tenderness will help to relieve the symptoms. It is important to make the injection correctly—injection directly into a tendon is associated with tendon rupture and injection into the subcutaneous tissue is associated with skin atrophy. Strict asepsis must be observed and up to three injections may be given at any one site at intervals of at least one month.

Rarely, epicondylitis is resistant to conservative treatment and surgical release of the tendinous aponeurosis is required.

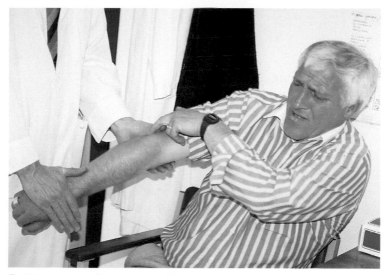

Fig. 62 Lateral epicondylar pain produced by resisted extension of the wrist.

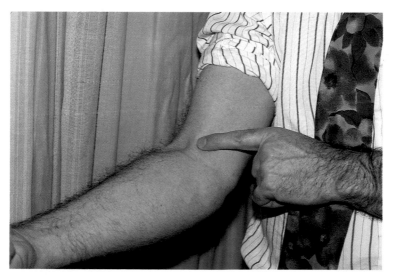

Fig. 63 Biceps tendinitis.

12 / The wrist

Colles fracture

A Colles fracture is produced by a fall on to the outstretched hand and occurs most commonly in elderly women. It results in a dinner-fork deformity of the wrist (Fig. 64).

Treatment   The need for reduction depends upon the position of the bone and the patient's age. Reduction may be under general or regional anaesthesia.

Bier's block. This is a simple technique (Fig. 65) which gives good regional anaesthesia using an appropriate local anaesthetic agent. A full pre-anaesthetic assessment should be made and the patient fasted as for a general anaesthetic. As with any regional anaesthetic technique, full resuscitation equipment must be available.

Swollen hand

Following injury, the hand may become markedly swollen. Resultant immobility of the hand and a dependent posture compound the swelling.

Treatment   The patient must have the limb elevated in a high arm sling and be encouraged to exercise the fingers and thumb at least once each hour.

Median nerve compression

This occurs usually secondarily to trauma or rheumatoid disease. The nerve is trapped in the carpal tunnel and causes pain in the hand and radial $3\frac{1}{2}$ digits with altered sensation in this area. Tinel's sign is positive (Fig. 66), i.e. tapping over the median nerve produces tingling within its distribution.

Treatment   Treatment may be conservative, by elevation of the limb, but surgical decompression may be required.

Rarely, median nerve compression may be associated with hypothyroidism or fluid retention in pregnancy. Treatment of the underlying thyroid disorder and the prescription of diuretics in pregnancy will relieve the symptoms.

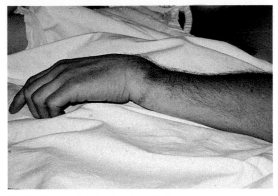

Fig. 64 Dinner-fork deformity of a Colles fracture.

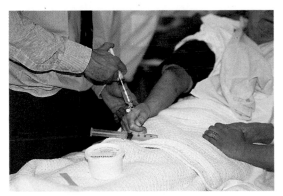

Fig. 65 Bier's block—note the double cuff.

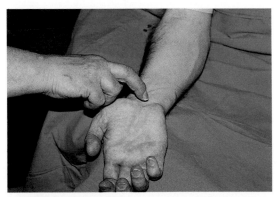

Fig. 66 Tinel's sign being elicited.

Lunate dislocation

This can dislocate alone or be associated with a fracture of the scaphoid and/or triquetral. The injury is usually missed if not specifically sought.

X-ray signs
- The abnormal spacing between the proximal carpal bones (Fig. 67).
- The triangular appearance of the lunate.
- The loss of the three crescents—the lunate sits in the crescent of the distal radius and the capitate sits in the crescent of the lunate (Fig. 68).

Smith's fracture

This occurs as a result of a fall on to the back of the hand. It is the reverse of a Colles fracture in that the distal fragment is angulated anteriorly (Fig. 69).

Treatment
Reduction is effected under anaesthesia with traction on the supinated forearm. A full arm cast is applied with the elbow at a right angle, the forearm in supination and the wrist dorsiflexed.

Fracture check-list

With any fracture, *always*:
- ascertain the mechanism of injury
- check whether there could be more than one injury
- examine the joint above and below the site of the injury.

In the forearm, don't forget the Galeazzi and Monteggia fracture–dislocations.

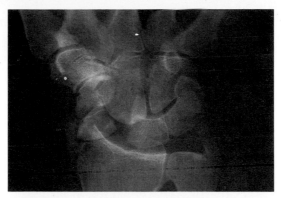

Fig. 67 Anteroposterior view of a perilunar dislocation.

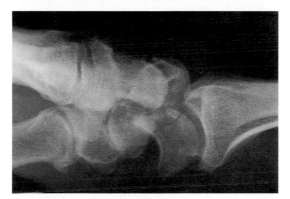

Fig. 68 Lateral view of a perilunar dislocation.

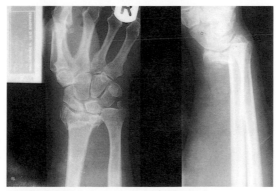

Fig. 69 A Smith's fracture.

Soft tissue conditions

Wrist sprains are common. They generally result from a hyperextension injury and can cause considerable discomfort which will persist for 4 to 6 weeks. The problem is to exclude a bony injury such as a scaphoid fracture.

Tenosynovitis

This term is used readily by patients, usually in relation to wrist pain secondary to unaccustomed repetitive activity such as home decorating or using a computer keyboard.

Tenosynovitis results from inflammation between the tendon and tendon sheath. The classical site is over the abductor pollicis longus and extensor pollicis brevis tendons on the radial side of the wrist. It may progress to tendon sheath stenosis—de Quervain's disease.

Clinical features There is swelling over the tendon (Fig. 70) and crepitation over the tendon sheath when the thumb is moved. Finkelstein's test (Fig. 71) involves the patient placing the thumb in the palm of the hand and gripping it by the fingers. Ulnar deviation of the hand produces pain.

Treatment Rest is very important and may be enforced by immobilization in a cast. If unsuccessful, a local steroid injection into the tendon sheath will help. Stenosis of the sheath requires surgical release.

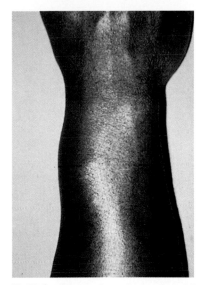

Fig. 70 Swelling over the tendons on the radial side of the wrist.

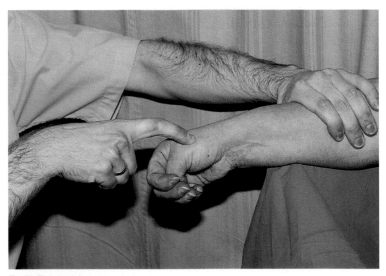

Fig. 71 Finkelstein's test.

The fractured scaphoid

Aetiology

This is due to a hyperextension injury, typically by falling on to the outstretched hand. It may occur in any age group but is most likely in young adult males.

Clinical features

There is tenderness in the anatomical snuffbox (Fig. 72), but it is important to palpate and compare tenderness in the right and left anatomical snuff boxes. Also palpate the dorsal and ventral aspects of the scaphoid to elicit tenderness (Fig. 73) and assess pain produced by axial compression of the thumb metacarpal on to the trapezium and thence the scaphoid (Fig. 74).

X-rays

These should be anteroposterior, lateral and the two 45° obliques. If a fracture is apparent radiologically, or any of the above diagnostic criteria are met, a forearm cast should be applied which immobilizes the thumb metacarpophalangeal joint. If a fracture is not confirmed, the cast should be removed at about 10 days and a further set of radiographs taken. Persisting tenderness and a normal second set of X-rays should be treated by further cast immobilization and a bone scan requested. This may give a definitive answer but care should be exercised in patients who exhibit arthritic changes at the base of the thumb since this can give a false positive result.

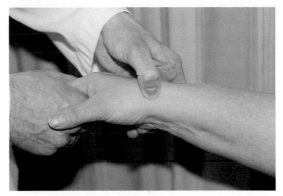

Fig. 72 Tenderness in the antomical snuff box.

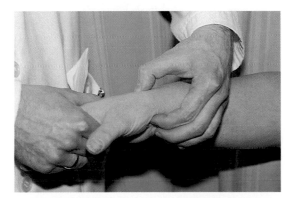

Fig. 73 Palpation of the dorsal and ventral surfaces of the scaphoid.

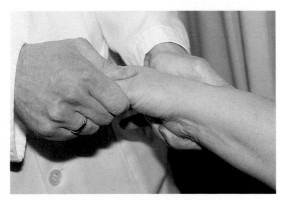

Fig. 74 Axial compression of the thumb.

13 / Hand conditions

Tendon injuries

Aetiology   A closed injury of the extensor tendon in the finger
disrupts the attachment of the extensor tendon on to the
middle or distal phalanx, causing a boutonnière or mallet
deformity respectively. A hyperextension injury may
avulse one of the flexor tendons or the volar plate at the
base of the middle phalanx.

Clinical features   ***Mallet finger*** (Fig. 75). This is associated with loss of
active extension of the distal interphalangeal joint.
X-rays may show an avulsed fragment of bone.

Boutonnière deformity (Fig. 76). This is due to the head
of the middle phalanx prolapsing dorsally between the
two slips of the extensor tendon and through the
extensor hood, producing the characteristic deformity.

Volar plate injuries. Injury to the volar plate produces
fusiform swelling, local pain and limitation of movement
at the proximal interphalangeal joint.

Open injuries. These do not necessarily produce a
characteristic posture or loss of function.

Treatment   • A boutonnière or mallet finger is treated
conservatively by splinting for 6 weeks (Fig. 77).
• Volar plate injuries are treated conservatively by
neighbour strapping for up to 2 weeks followed by
active mobilization.
• Open injuries to the tendons must be suspected when
presented with any wound on the wrist or hand. It is
important to assess the function of all deep structures.
If there is any doubt, referral to a hand surgeon must
be made.

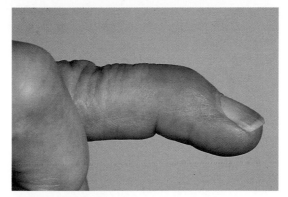

Fig. 75 A mallet deformity.

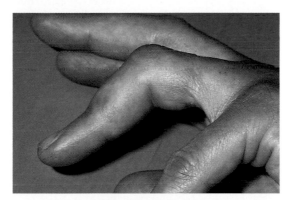

Fig. 76 A boutonnière deformity.

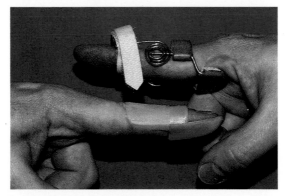

Fig. 77 A Capener and mallet splint.

Nail injuries

Aetiology

The major cause of injury to the nail and distal phalanx is a crush injury. Less commonly, direct wounds are responsible.

Clinical features

A subungual haematoma (Fig. 78) may be associated with a fracture of the distal phalanx. It is exquisitely tender and X-rays reveal any associated fracture.

Dislocation of the nail root from beneath the cuticle (Fig. 79) may also be associated with a fracture of the distal phalanx. The fracture is typically transverse with anterior angulation of the distal fragment.

Treatment

Subungual haematoma. The haematoma is drained by a small hole drilled through the nail. The hole may be made with a red-hot paper clip, a sterile hypodermic needle or a commercially available drill. Early evacuation of liquid blood is much more effective in relieving pain than attempted later evacuation of semi-clotted blood. If there is a fracture, antibiotics should be given.

Dislocated nail. The nail should be replaced carefully (Fig. 80) for two reasons: firstly to act as a splint for the distal bony fragment and to hold the distal soft tissues in place and secondly to prevent damage to the developing nail caused by adhesions between the cuticle and germinal part of the nail bed (Fig. 81).

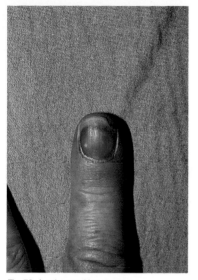

Fig. 78 A subungual haematoma.

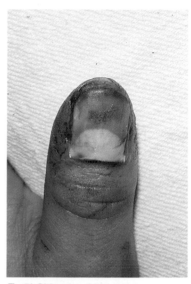

Fig. 79 Dislocation of the nail root.

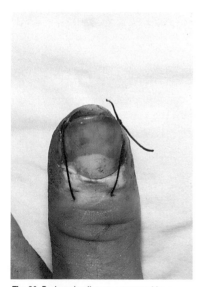

Fig. 80 Reduced nail root, supported by a horizontal mattress suture.

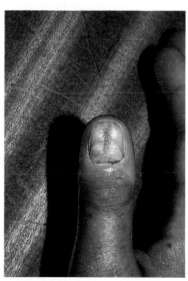

Fig. 81 Ridging of the nail resulting from damage to the germinal epithelium.

Fingertip injuries

Aetiology Full thickness skin loss from the tip of the finger or thumb may be caused by either a sharp or blunt injury.

Treatment **Incomplete amputation.** The fingertip may be reconstructed carefully using either steristrips or lightly placed sutures and has a good chance of survival, particularly in children.

Complete amputation (Fig. 82). This requires tissue cover. If bone is proud of the soft tissue, the patient should be referred for definitive surgery but, if the bone is not proud, it can be managed in the accident and emergency department. Replantation may be considered, particularly if the amputation has been caused by a clean, incised injury rather than a tearing, crush injury. It is most likely to be attempted in one of the radial three digits because of their importance to the grip.

Surgical cover by means of a skin graft may be used but this often creates a fingertip with markedly impaired sensation, an obviously deformed fingertip (Fig. 83) and an obvious, initially very painful, graft donor site (Fig. 84) which leaves a permanent scar.

Conservative treatment, using silver sulphadiazine cream or a non-adherent tulle-gras dressing, allows spontaneous healing within 4 to 6 weeks. This produces a cosmetically good result, the sensation of the tip returns to near normal, and it avoids the scar of a graft donor site.

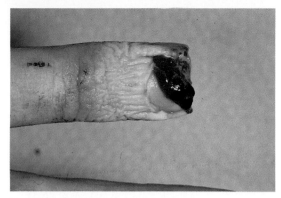

Fig. 82 Complete amputation of the fingertip.

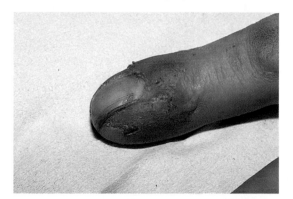

Fig. 83 Previously amputated fingertip treated by grafting. Note the nail spike.

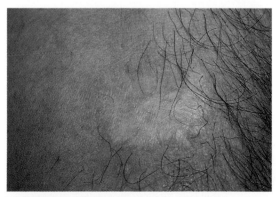

Fig. 84 Graft donor site from same source as Figure 83.

Infections

Aetiology

These may develop as a primary infection but more commonly occur secondary to a trivial wound or retained foreign body. The infecting organisms include streptococci and staphylococci but a wide variety of other organisms may be seen, particularly in butchers or gardeners.

Clinical features

There is marked swelling resulting from the inflammatory oedema occurring in an area where the tissue is very lax. Pyogenic infection may produce a collection of pus in one of the deep palmar spaces (Fig. 85) and there may be lymphangitis and systemic upset.

Following a relatively minor injury, there may be the sinister complication of flexor tendon sheath infection associated with tissue necrosis (Fig. 86). This is characterized by exquisitely painful active or passive movement of the affected finger, with tenderness along the flexor tendon proximal to the site of obvious infection.

Treatment

This involves elevation of the limb, high dose antibiotics and frequent review.

If there is systemic upset or clinical evidence of any pus collection in a palmar space or tendon sheath, urgent decompression must be undertaken to prevent damage to the palmar structures or fibrous adhesions to the tendon.

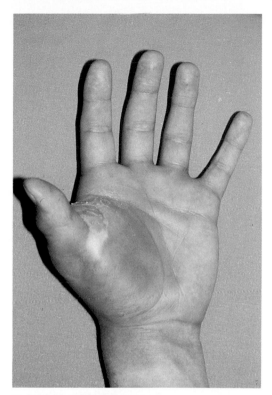

Fig. 85 Pyogenic infection in the hand.

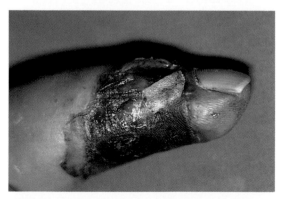

Fig. 86 Skin infection and necrosis resulting from deep-seated infection.

Miscellaneous problems

Degloving
injuries

These result from catching the hand in machinery or catching a ring on something (Fig. 87). The ring cuts into the soft tissue at the base of the finger and tears it distally. There is impairment of the neurovascular function and the underlying tendon or bone may be damaged. Early referral to a hand unit is indicated since microsurgery might be contemplated if the degree of nerve and vessel damage is not too great.

Fractures

Non-displaced fractures of the fingers or hand are usually treated conservatively by neighbour strapping or resting in a cast. However, even with apparently 'non-displaced' fractures, it is important to check that there has been no rotation of the metacarpal or phalanx and, if present, this should be corrected prior to immobilization. If this is not undertaken there may be significant functional disability caused by overlapping of the digits when the patient makes a fist (Fig. 89).

High pressure
injection

High pressure oil, paint or air injection into a digit is an apparently innocuous injury (Fig. 88) but must be treated urgently. The foreign material passes for a surprisingly great distance into the digit and requires early surgical evacuation of the foreign material and débridement of damaged tissue. The injected oil or paint is very irritant to the tissues and may also result in impairment of the circulation.

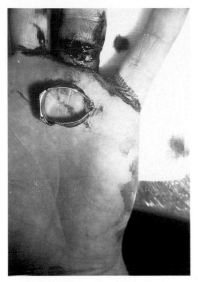

Fig. 87 Ring injury to a finger.

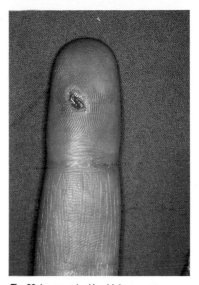

Fig. 88 Innocent-looking high pressure injection site.

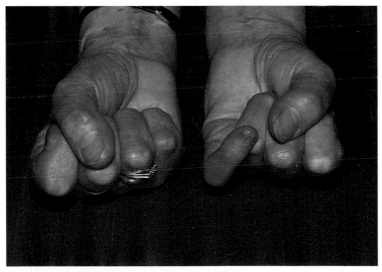

Fig. 89 Rotation of the little finger secondary to a spiral fracture.

14 / **Perianal conditions**

Aetiology
- *Haemorrhoids* are dilated veins of a plexus at and below the anorectal ring. They are of unknown aetiology but are more common in postpartum females.
- *Perianal haematoma*, occurring usually spontaneously.
- *Fissure-in-ano*, a tear in the anal mucosa which results in painful spasm of the anal sphincter.
- *Threadworm infection* in children.

Symptoms
These include pain, pruritus and spotting of blood on the underwear. Haemorrhoids may enlarge and be extruded through the anus and may be classified as first, second or third degree, depending on the propensity with which they prolapse and the ease with which they can be reduced (Fig. 90). A perianal haematoma causes a localized, tender swelling at the anal margin. Threadworms cause irritation at night when they lay their eggs in the perianal region.

Treatment
Third degree (irreducible) haemorrhoids: cause considerable local pain and may bleed, ulcerate or thrombose. This is a surgical emergency and should be treated either by reduction or excision under general anaesthesia.

Perianal haematoma: relieved instantly by incision and evacuation.

Fissure-in-ano: treatment usually involves stretching of the anal sphincter under general anaesthesia, or a lateral anal sphincterotomy.

Threadworms (Fig. 91): respond to oral medication, such as piperazine or mebendazole.

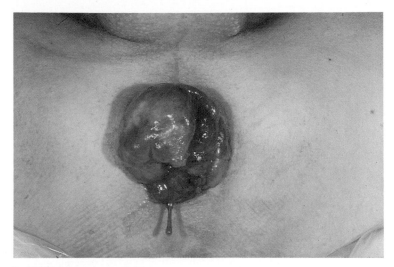

Fig. 90 Third degree haemorrhoids.

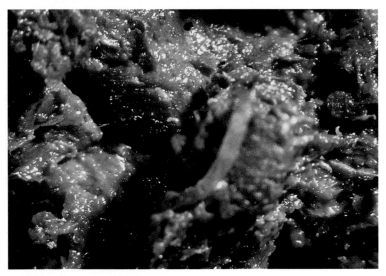

Fig. 91 Threadworm on a specimen of faeces.

Infective conditions

Aetiology
- This is usually secondary to infection of a hair follicle or secondary to trauma to the mucosa of the anal canal (Fig. 92).
- A pilonidal sinus is one which is related to an area of skin which has been irritated by hair. Typically, it occurs over the lower sacrum or coccyx (Fig. 93), but may also occur on the hand, such as that of a hairdresser.

Symptoms
Pain is of a deep, throbbing nature and increases when sitting or straining to evacuate the bowels. There may be systemic upset with pyrexia and tachycardia, and this may also lead to septicaemia. Infection may track along the portal circulation leading to portal pyaemia and a liver abscess.

A pilonidal sinus is associated with local discomfort, a moist discharge and recurrent abscess formation.

Treatment
Early drainage of an ischiorectal or perianal abscess, usually under antibiotic cover, should be undertaken and a careful examination carried out under anaesthetic lest a fistula or sinus should be missed.

A pilonidal abscess should be drained surgically but, in the absence of an abscess, the track should be opened and allowed to granulate. Alternatively, the sinus should be excised fully and a primary closure obtained.

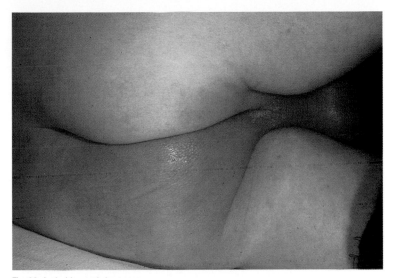

Fig. 92 An ischiorectal abscess.

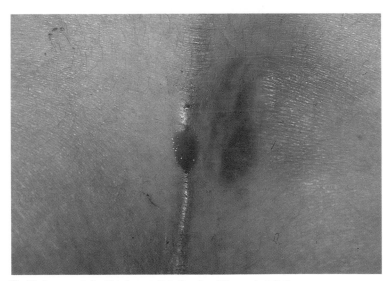

Fig. 93 A recurrent pilonidal abscess. Note the pit and the purulent discharge.

Foreign bodies

Aetiology Ingested foreign bodies may become lodged in the rectum; alternatively, they may be introduced from below during sexual activity and are usually phallic in shape. Occasionally, they may be accidental in aetiology (Fig. 94).

Clinical features There may be features of intestinal obstruction or pain in the perineum. X-rays confirm the presence of the foreign material and exclude complications such as perforation of the bowel. Digital rectal examination should be done carefully lest the material should be pushed beyond reach.

Treatment If introduced from above (Fig. 95), foreign material is most likely to impact in the upper oesophagus, at the pylorus or at the ileocaecal valve. If it is in the rectum, it is likely to pass spontaneously.

Foreign bodies introduced from below slip beyond the anal sphincter and into the rectum. Digital removal may be possible (Fig. 96), but this often proves difficult because of discomfort and inability to grasp the object. General anaesthesia allows full relaxation, dilatation of the anal sphincter and removal via a sigmoidoscope or colonoscope.

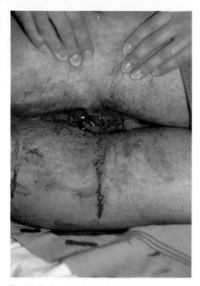

Fig. 94 Perianal wound resulting from impalement on a 14 cm spike.

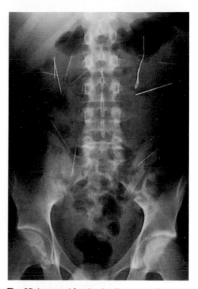

Fig. 95 Ingested foreign bodies—spot the razor blade.

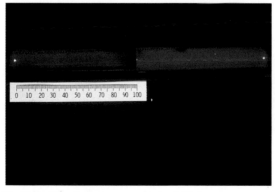

Fig. 96 Rectal foreign body removed in the A & E department.

15 / Genitourinary problems

Paraphimosis

Aetiology The tight prepuce becomes trapped behind the engorged glans penis and each becomes further swollen (Fig. 97). The patient is usually a young adult who is reluctant to seek help and any delay in seeking treatment makes the problem worse due to venous engorgement.

Treatment Application of an ice pack may allow the swelling to reduce sufficiently to allow reduction but an alternative is to inject hyaluronidase and local anaesthetic into the constricting band prior to reduction.

Wounds

Aetiology Frenular tears can occur, usually during sexual intercourse. The frenal artery may be torn and this causes dramatic bleeding.

Treatment It may be necessary to under-run and ligate the artery but it is seldom necessary to suture the wound which heals without any problem.

Genital infections

The significance of these conditions to an accident and emergency department is to identify them and refer them to an appropriate unit without giving treatment which might mask specialist tests. The most common infections seen are non-specific urethritis, gonorrhoea (Fig. 98) and herpetic infections (Fig. 99). This latter condition is often very painful and may lead to acute retention of urine and the patient may require admission to the hospital.

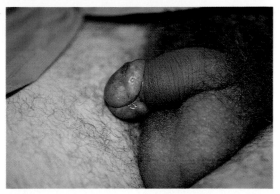

Fig. 97 A paraphimosis.

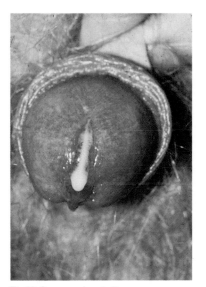

Fig. 98 Gonococcal urethritis.

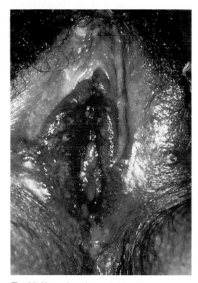

Fig. 99 Herpetic vulvovaginitis.

Urethral trauma

This must be suspected whenever there has been major trauma resulting in a pelvic fracture (Fig. 100) or trauma involving the perineum. The diagnosis would be suggested by perineal or scrotal haematoma (Fig. 101), blood at the external urethral meatus or a high-riding prostate on digital rectal examination. Urethral catheterization must not be attempted and all such cases must be referred for a urological opinion (Fig. 102).

The fractured pelvis

Diagnosis   Instability or pain with pelvic springing are not reliable signs of a pelvic fracture. It should be suspected in all cases of major trauma and appropriate radiographs taken.

Treatment   Blood loss into the loose pelvic tissues and retroperitoneal space can be very substantial so adequate intravenous fluid should be given and this includes a blood transfusion. Urgent reduction and fixation of displaced fractures should be undertaken, particularly if there is clinical evidence of continued haemorrhage. If urgent surgery is necessary and there is any delay which jeopardizes the patient's condition, a MAST suit (military anti-shock trousers) may be applied to gain time but this should be the exception rather than the rule.

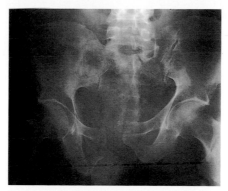

Fig. 100 Fracture–separation of the symphysis pubis and left sacroiliac joint.

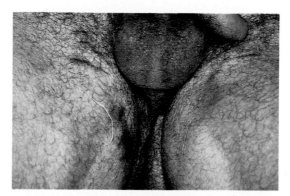

Fig. 101 Perineal bruising resulting from falling astride a blunt object.

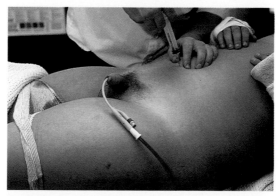

Fig. 102 Suspected urethral injury catheterized safely by a urologist.

Urine retention

Aetiology   This can present due to prostatic obstruction or blood clot from a bladder lesion such as a papilloma. More commonly, it results from blockage of an indwelling catheter (Fig. 103) in a patient referred from the community.

Clinical features   There is a painfully swollen bladder, often with overflow incontinence. 'Chronic' retention usually presents with painless bladder distension and overflow.

Treatment   Local policy will dictate whether the urologist or A & E staff performs the catheterization. Whenever it is done, it is important to use a full aseptic technique and arrange for formal review in order to diagnose and treat the underlying pathology.

Retention in women is uncommon and is usually due to a neurological disorder, pelvic obstruction by an ovarian cyst, tumour or by herpes simplex vulvitis.

Testicular torsion

This is a true emergency. The age group is between puberty and the late twenties.

Clinical features   There is acute onset of lower abdominal pain with testicular discomfort. The testis is swollen (Fig. 104) and tender and there is thickening of the vas deferens.
    The differential diagnosis is from epididymo-orchitis.

Treatment   Urgent ultrasonography, followed by surgery if the diagnosis is confirmed.

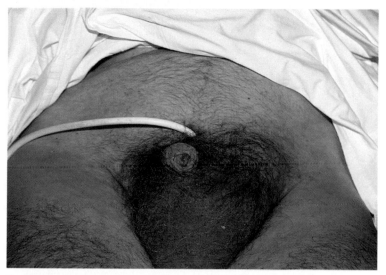

Fig. 103 Long-term indwelling suprapubic catheter. Note the left inguinal hernia.

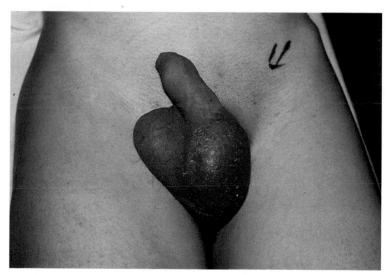

Fig. 104 4-day-old torsion of the left testis.

16 / **Hip pain**

Aetiology   Fracture of the femoral neck occurs most commonly in the elderly as a result of minor trauma, or in patients with porotic bones. The differential diagnosis is from a fracture of the pubic rami. Other causes include exacerbation of degenerative disease and dislocation of the hip or a prosthesis.

Clinical features   There is pain in the hip and difficulty bearing weight. The posture of the limb gives evidence of the diagnosis: a patient presenting with a fracture of the femoral neck has external rotation of the limb because of spasm in the psoas major and there is shortening of the limb (Fig. 105) whilst, in one who has dislocated the hip, there is adduction, internal rotation and flexion at the hip (Fig. 106). Active and passive movements of the hip are painful. Fracture of the pubic rami produces no abnormal posture. Pelvic springing may be painful and, if extensive or grossly displaced, the fracture may result in hypovolaemia or damage to the bladder or urethra.

    X-rays of the pelvis and hip are necessary to confirm the clinical diagnosis.

Treatment   Referral for admission to hospital is usually necessary. Non-displaced fractures of the pubic rami can be treated at home with analgesia providing there is sufficient social support.

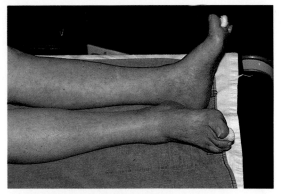

Fig. 105 Fracture of the right femoral neck.

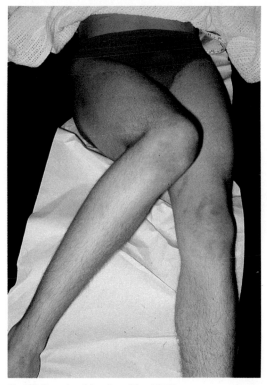

Fig. 106 Posterior dislocation of the right hip.

17 / The groin

Anatomy The inguinal ligament is not a ligament in the strict sense but the lower free margin of the external oblique aponeurosis. It spans the interval between the anterior superior iliac spine and pubic tubercle. Structures passing deep to the ligament include the femoral neurovascular bundle, the musculotendinous units of psoas and iliacus and also loose connective tissue and lymphatics in the femoral canal.

Clinical relevance The femoral artery is the key structure in the region and it lies halfway between the anterior superior iliac spine and the pubic symphysis, lying medial to the mid-inguinal point. The femoral vein and nerve lie 1 centimetre medially and laterally respectively. The neurovascular bundle lies superficially and may be damaged easily ('butcher's thigh'—Fig. 107). Do not explore wounds in the A & E department but refer the patient to an appropriate surgeon for formal exploration in theatre.

Venous and arterial blood can be drawn easily or the vein cannulated by direct puncture or cut down on to the great saphenous vein which drains into the femoral vein just distal to the groin skin crease.

Femoral nerve block
This is of great benefit in the management of a fracture of the femoral shaft, patellar dislocation and some femoral neck fractures. The local anaesthetic solution is infiltrated in all directions around the nerve (Fig. 108) to produce profound analgesia. This obviates the need for opiates.

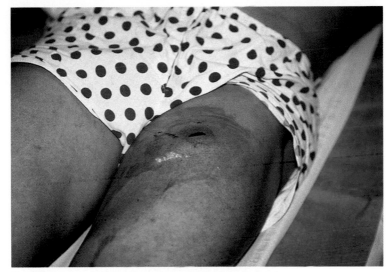

Fig. 107 Damage to the femoral vessels resulting from a stab wound.

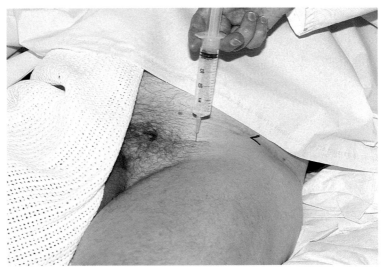

Fig. 108 A femoral nerve block.

18 / **The knee**

General injury

History
The mechanism of injury may give essential clues as to the likely injury but the speed of the incident is often so great that the patient cannot remember the details.

Rapid swelling of the joint (within an hour) is likely to be due to a haemarthrosis (Fig. 109). This is very painful and is due to damage to bone, or to capsular or ligamentous structures.

Swelling developing more slowly is likely to be due to synovial irritation. The swelling is not tense or particularly painful.

Investigation
Clinical examination is the most important. Plain X-rays may show the presence of an obvious fracture but the presence of a lipohaemarthrosis (Fig. 110) is pathognomonic of an intra-articular fracture. This is seen on the lateral film with a horizontal beam as a layer of less dense fat floating on more dense blood in the suprapatellar pouch.

Treatment
A tense haemarthrosis should be aspirated under strict aseptic conditions. If done under anaesthesia, examination of the ligamentous structures can be assessed fully.

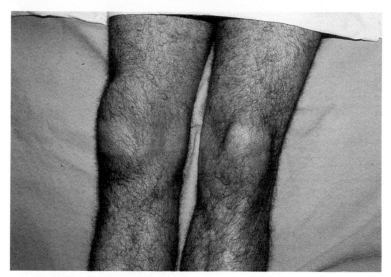

Fig. 109 A haemarthrosis in the right knee.

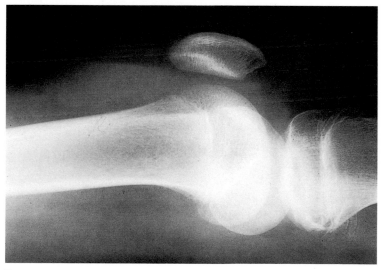

Fig. 110 A lipohaemarthrosis—note the horizontal fat/blood fluid level.

Ligament injuries

History A varus or valgus force may suggest a collateral ligament injury. Paradoxically, a complete rupture produces little pain or swelling.

Clinical features A patient with a partial tear will have pain when bearing weight, whilst a complete rupture may cause little disability if walking steadily in a straight line. Varus and valgus stability is afforded by both the collateral and cruciate ligaments. If a collateral ligament injury is suspected, the joint must be stressed in a position of 30° flexion since, in the extended position, intact cruciate ligaments can account for apparently full stability (Fig. 111).

Cruciate ligament stability is tested in a position of 90° flexion and an attempt made to draw the upper tibia forwards and backwards (Fig. 112). Instability of the anterior and posterior ligament respectively, is suggested by increased displacement compared with the normal side.

Treatment Injuries to the ligaments require referral to an orthopaedic surgeon. Less severe injuries will be immobilized initially in a cylinder cast whilst more severe injuries may require surgical intervention.

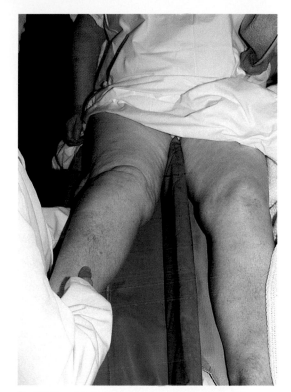

Fig. 111 Complete rupture of the medial collateral and both cruciate ligaments.

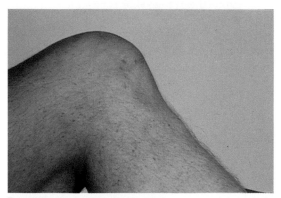

Fig. 112 Positive posterior drawer sign due to a torn posterior cruciate ligament.

Anterior knee pain

Ruptured quadriceps

This occurs mainly in the older age group as a result of a fall.

Clinical features   There is local tenderness and a gap in the tendon is palpable just above the patella (Fig. 113). It is confirmed by the inability to extend the knee against gravity or lift the foot clear from the couch.

Treatment   Treatment is operative.

Patellar dislocation

Aetiology   The patella dislocates laterally (Fig. 114) because of the direction of action of the quadriceps muscle and the relatively shallow lateral femoral condyle. A small, high-lying patella predisposes to dislocation which occurs most commonly in young women.

Clinical features   Most patients will relocate the patella before they attend hospital so the diagnosis relies upon the history, local swelling, and a positive apprehension test. This is a concerned expression and contraction of the quadriceps if the patella is subluxed laterally.

X-rays must include a skyline view to identify a marginal patellar or femoral condylar fracture.

Treatment   Treatment is conservative by immobilization in a cylinder cast following aspiration of the effusion if it is tense.

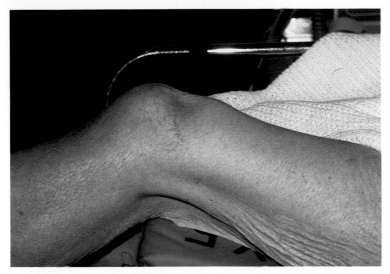

Fig. 113 Rupture of the quadriceps tendon.

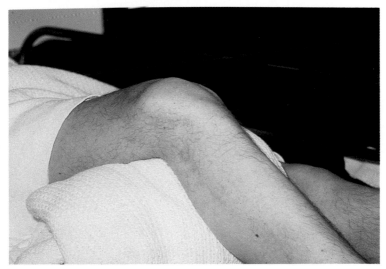

Fig. 114 Lateral dislocation of the right patella.

Quadriceps wasting

Patients who have sustained an injury to the knee may rapidly develop wasting of the quadriceps muscle (Fig. 115). All such patients must be given instruction on quadriceps exercises to maintain the muscle bulk since this has an important stabilizing function of both the knee and patellofemoral joint. The clinical entity of a knee which 'gives way' is due to transient loss of power in the quadriceps muscle and is a reflex phenomenon, resulting most commonly from chondromalacia patellae, entrapment of a synovial fold, a loose body or a torn meniscus.

The locked knee

Get a clear history. True locking is the terminal loss of extension (Fig. 116) and the block is firm rather than spongy.

Aetiology There is a mechanical block due to a fragment of a torn meniscus, or a loose body, resulting from trauma or osteochondritis dissecans. The fragment floats into the joint between the femoral and tibial condyles and causes the mechanical block. The block often resolves spontaneously because the fragment floats into the suprapatellar pouch.

Treatment A patient with a locked knee requires admission for examination under anaesthesia, followed by arthroscopy and removal of the loose fragment. Alternatively, the loose fragment can be visualized by radiography such as magnetic resonance imaging techniques.

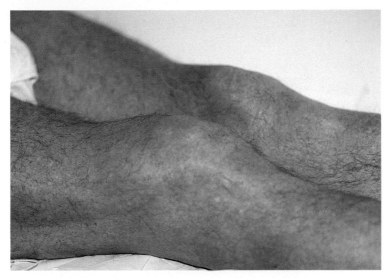

Fig. 115 Quadriceps wasting of the right thigh associated with a knee effusion.

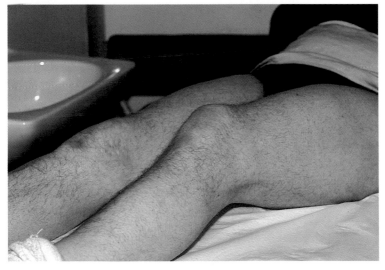

Fig. 116 Inability to fully extend the knee.

19 / **The leg**

Varicose veins

These are dilated, tortuous subcutaneous veins which occur most commonly in the postpartum period (Fig. 117).

Clinical features   They cause aching locally and can bleed torrentially following minor trauma. Longstanding varicose veins produce distal ischaemic changes in the skin and subcutaneous tissue, particularly around the medial malleolus. Trauma may produce an ulcer which is resistant to treatment (Fig. 118).

Treatment   **Haemorrhage**: elevation of the limb and direct pressure over the bleeding point.

Ulcers: application of a non-adherent dressing, a firm support from toes to knee and advice regarding elevation of the limb.

Muscular pain

- Acute partial tears of the calf muscles occur most commonly in young and middle-aged adults during exertion (Fig. 119). There is local tenderness, swelling and bruising.
- A compartment syndrome following trauma or exertion results from increased pressure within one of the muscle sheaths. It produces tenderness of the muscle, pain when the muscle is stretched and, later, there is evidence of neurovascular compression.
- Spontaneous onset of calf pain raises the suspicion of a deep vein thrombosis.

Treatment   A heel raise reduces the tension in the gastrocnemius complex and elevation helps to reduce swelling of the calf muscles. A compartment syndrome should be referred to the orthopaedic surgeon. Exclude a deep venous thrombosis by investigations such as venography.

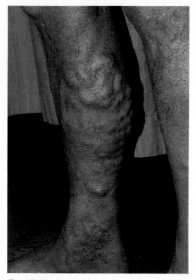

Fig. 117 Varicose veins.

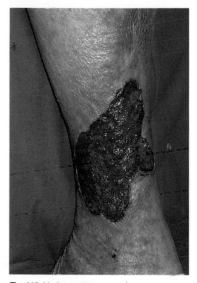

Fig. 118 Varicose ulcer secondary to trauma.

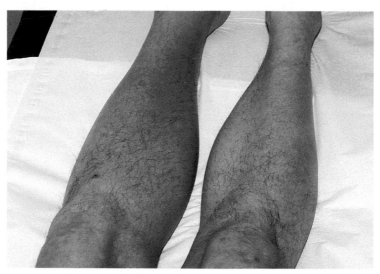

Fig. 119 Partial tear of the left gastrocnemius resulting in bruising.

20 / **The ankle**

Ligamentous injury

Anatomy

The lateral ligament of the ankle is divided into three parts which pass forwards, downwards and backwards from the lateral malleolus. An inversion sprain causes tearing of the anterior fibres, whilst a more severe injury is associated with progressive tearing of the middle and posterior fibres which can result in instability of the joint.

Clinical features

There is marked swelling and tenderness over the lateral aspect of the ankle. Careful clinical examination does not exclude bony injury so X-rays should be taken. It is important to assess the medial aspect of the joint as well as the whole of the leg, since injuries to these areas may also occur in conjunction with an apparently isolated sprain of the lateral ligament. There may be alarming bruising which tracks along the lateral border of the foot and under the sole of the foot (Figs 120 & 121). This may itself cause an irritant synovitis of the small joints of the foot. If there is any question of ligamentous instability, stress X-rays (Fig. 122) should be performed under anaesthetic and the stability of each ankle compared.

Treatment

This is aimed at reducing the swelling and improving mobility of the ankle and subtalar complex. Rest, strapping, ice and elevation are advised and the patient is encouraged to walk as normally as possible.

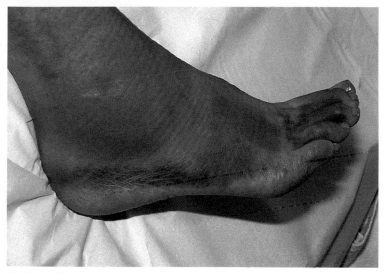

Fig. 120 Swelling and bruising from a sprain of the lateral ligament.

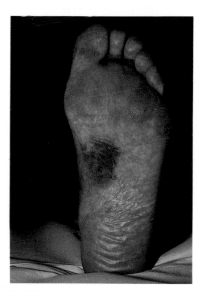

Fig. 121 Bruising on the sole of the foot, tracking from the lateral ligament.

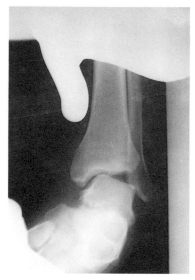

Fig. 122 Stress X-ray showing instability of the lateral ligament complex.

Bone and joint conditions

An extensive injury (Fig. 123) to the soft tissues or bones around the ankle may lead to dislocation or subluxation of the ankle or subtalar complex. The foot is usually displaced laterally and rotated externally relative to the leg. Reduction must be effected as a matter of urgency to prevent traction injuries to the neurovascular structures and also to minimize ischaemic damage to the skin which is under tension over the malleolus. Less extensive injuries such as fractures of the lateral malleolus (Fig. 124) are more common and often associated with sport.

Rupture of the Achilles tendon

The Achilles tendon is the combined tendinous structures of the gastrocnemius and soleus muscles. It attaches distally on to the posterior surface of the calcaneum.

Aetiology   Rupture of the Achilles tendon (Fig. 125) occurs most often in middle-aged men and results from physical exertion. The patient feels sudden pain over the tendon and this may be accompanied by an audible snap.

Clinical features   When seen early, there may be an easily palpable gap but, when seen later, the gap is indistinct because of haemorrhage and inflammatory oedema. When the calf is squeezed gently with the patient prone, the foot does not plantarflex to the same extent as the normal side (Simmond's test).

Treatment   Treatment may be conservative or operative and should be dictated by the preferences of the local orthopaedic surgeons.

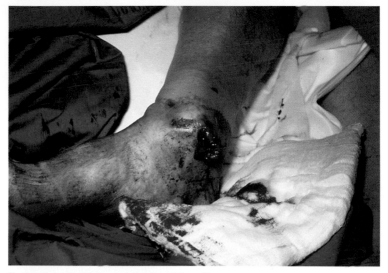

Fig. 123 Compound fracture–dislocation of the ankle.

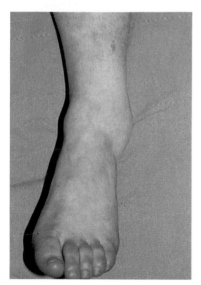

Fig. 124 Fracture of the lateral malleolus.

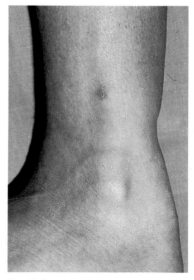

Fig. 125 Ruptured Achilles tendon.

21 / **Bursitis**

Anatomy   A bursa is a synovial sac which is a protective mechanism preventing damage to soft tissues by pressure on a bony surface. Bursae occur typically over bony prominences but may occur also in relation to tendons or ligaments at major joints (Figs 126 & 127).

Aetiology   Inflammation is most commonly sterile and related to a repetitive occupational activity (Fig. 128). Occasionally, the bursitis may be infective and associated with an abrasion or an episode of septicaemia. Rarely, the bursitis may be gouty or rheumatoid in origin.

Clinical features   The area shows the cardinal features of acute inflammation, heat, redness, pain and loss of movement and there may also be crepitus. There is usually no associated lymphatic involvement and aspiration of the bursa reveals pale yellow serous fluid. Infective, gouty or rheumatoid bursitis is associated with turbid, thick aspirate and laboratory examination of the fluid may be very helpful in confirming the diagnosis.

Treatment   Sterile bursitis is treated by rest, support, local ice pack and non-steroidal anti-inflammatory agents. If non-infective bursitis has not responded to this treatment, it may be treated by aspiration and instillation of a locally acting steroid. Infective bursitis should be drained surgically and the other unusual causes should be treated by a rheumatologist.

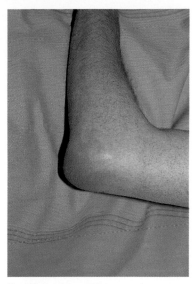

Fig. 126 An olecranon bursa.

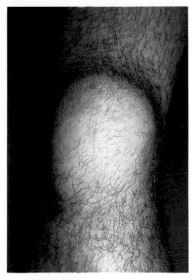

Fig. 127 Prepatellar bursa (housemaid's knee).

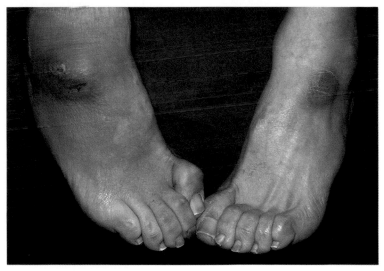

Fig. 128 Occupational bursitis in a tailor.

22 / Skin conditions

Virus infections

Herpes zoster

This is due to varicella zoster virus which emerges from posterior roots of the spinal nerves and the sensory cranial nerves.

Clinical features   There is prodromal pain which can mimic visceral pain such as a myocardial infarction. After a few days, redness of the skin develops and vesicles appear within a particular dermatome (Fig. 129).

Treatment   Acyclovir may be used to treat the skin lesions. Sufficiently strong analgesia is important.

Herpes simplex

Clinical features   This is subdivided into type I, which is associated predominantly with oral lesions (cold sores), and type II, which is associated predominantly with genital lesions, but this rule is not always true. Occasionally, the virus can affect the corneal epithelium to produce a dendritic ulcer (see also Fig. 25, p. 20 & Fig. 99, p. 74).

Treatment   Early treatment with acyclovir ointment can reduce the severity of the lesions.

Warts

Clinical features   These are common and found mainly on the hands (Fig. 130). They are spread by direct contact and may be painful if present on the feet.

Treatment   Treatment may be by topical salicylic acid or cryotherapy with liquid nitrogen.

Molluscum contagiosum

Clinical features   An unusual condition which presents with clusters of painless discrete pearly raised lesions without any surrounding erythema (Fig. 131).

Treatment   Treatment is by pricking the centre of each with a sharpened wooden stick which has been dipped in phenol solution or betadine.

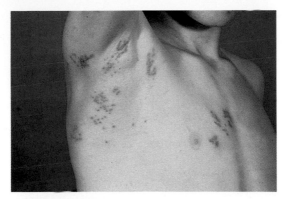

Fig. 129 Herpes zoster.

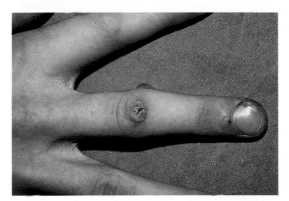

Fig. 130 Warts.

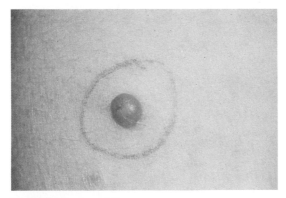

Fig. 131 Molluscum contagiosum.

Miscellaneous conditions

Eczema

Aetiology   This is usually allergic in nature but may also be due to atopy. Allergic eczema may be due to medication, plants, animals or cosmetics. Jewellery, particularly items containing nickel, produces characteristic patterns of eczema (Fig. 132).

Clinical features   Eczema presents as an itchy rash which forms vesicles and these break down and become encrusted.

Treatment   Referral to a dermatologist should be made in order to identify any definite allergens and to advise about prevention of further problems.

Topical steroids are used. Care must be taken regarding the strength of the steroid, particularly if they are used on the face, as skin atrophy and telangiectasia can result. If there is a superadded infection, a topical antibiotic may be used in conjunction with the steroid.

Pityriasis rosea

This can be an alarming rash with a 'herald patch' (Fig. 133) which is the first sign of the rash to appear. It is large, oval and has a scaly margin. Subsequently, further smaller lesions develop and these tend to be arranged in a horizontal line. The rash is self-limiting over a period of between 4 and 6 weeks.

Lichen planus

The patient may present with flat-topped, multiangular lesions which are shiny and violaceous. They are common on the flexor aspect of the wrists and may be itchy. White striations are seen on the buccal mucosa (Fig. 134).

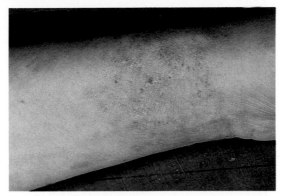

Fig. 132 Allergy to a nickel bracelet.

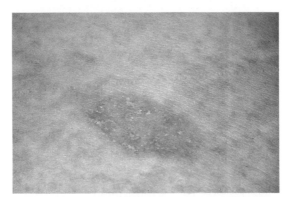

Fig. 133 Herald patch in pityriasis rosea.

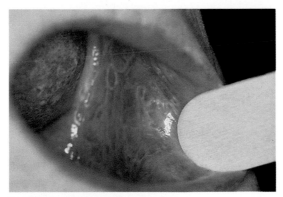

Fig. 134 Buccal mucosa in lichen planus.

Tumours

It is important to identify those lesions which may be
readily removed without risk and to be able to identify
those lesions which should be referred to a dermatologist
as they may be malignant.

Clinical types **Melanoma**. This is usually a dark, pigmented lesion with
an irregular border. There may be the history of a pre-
existing mole which has increased recently in size, may
have bled, ulcerated or become itchy. Beware of the
subungual melanoma (Fig. 135) which may inadvertently
be explored as an infection or haematoma.

Rodent ulcer. This is a basal cell carcinoma which occurs
most commonly on the face (Fig. 136). It has a raised,
shiny edge and dilated blood vessels may cross this edge.
Although it does not metastasize, it is locally very
invasive.

Squamous cell carcinoma. This is a hard nodule which
may appear warty (Fig. 137). Larger lesions ulcerate
and metastasis is not uncommon. Treatment is by local
excision or radiotherapy.

Keratoacanthoma. This is a rapidly growing, benign
skin tumour which may ulcerate (Fig. 138). It may
resemble a squamous cell carcinoma histologically but
the rapid growth and spontaneous resolution are
pathognomonic.

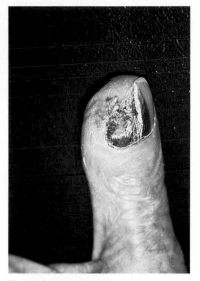

Fig. 135 Subungual melanoma.

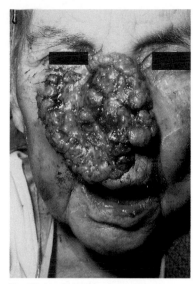

Fig. 136 Locally invasive rodent ulcer.

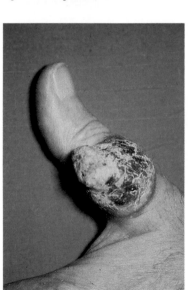

Fig. 137 A squamous cell carcinoma presenting as a wart.

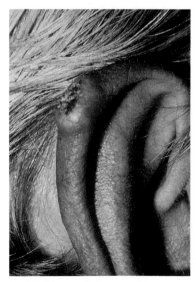

Fig. 138 A keratoacanthoma.

23 / Soft tissue infection

Aetiology **Cellulitis** (Fig. 139): a rapidly spreading infection of subcutaneous tissue caused most often by *Streptococcus pyogenes*. It may be haematogenous or introduced by an apparently insignificant wound.

Pyogenic infection: may develop de novo or in a pre-existing cyst (Fig. 140). The most common organism is *Staphylococcus aureus* and an abscess may develop anywhere but the most common sites are the breast, axilla and ischiorectal fossa.

Clinical features Cellulitis produces an area which is red, warm, tender and swollen and there may be features of systemic upset with fever and tachycardia. In addition, a pyogenic infection presents a localized fluctuant swelling.

Treatment **Cellulitis**: treated with high dose antibiotics and the patient reviewed daily. If systemic upset is a prominent feature, admission to hospital is advised and intravenous antibiotics given.

Pyogenic infection: the abscess can be treated by opening with a cruciate incision and trimming off the corners (Fig. 141). This ensures that the skin wound does not heal before the cavity becomes obliterated with granulation tissue. Alternatively, the cavity can be curetted and packed loosely with paraffin gauze or obliterated with large mattress sutures. If the latter is undertaken, a loading dose of antibiotic is given pre-operatively or antibiotic cream may be injected into the cavity.

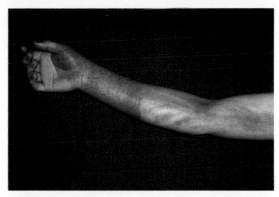

Fig. 139 Cellulitis with lymphangitis—the 'red lines of death'.

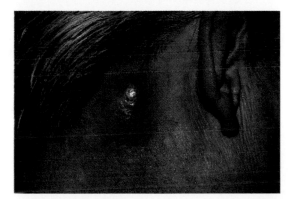

Fig. 140 Infected sebaceous cyst.

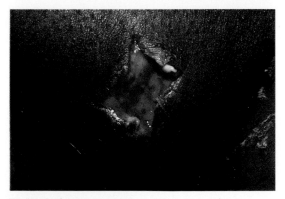

Fig. 141 Cruciate incision to treat an abscess on the buttock.

Pyogenic granuloma

This is a small nodule of granulation tissue which occurs most commonly on the fingers following minor trauma. It grows slowly and there is no associated cellulitis.

Treatment Thorough curettage should be performed and the specimen sent for histological confirmation. Small recurrences may be cauterized with silver nitrate or liquid nitrogen (Fig. 142).

Paronychia

An infection of the nail fold may track proximally beneath the cuticle or the nail (Fig. 143).

Treatment Early treatment with antibiotics may prevent the formation of pus but it often requires drainage over the area of maximum fluctuation or by opening the interval between the nail and cuticle. If the nail is floating freely, it should be removed completely.

Ingrowing toenails

These occur commonly in adolescent or young adult males, and affect the nail folds (Fig. 144).

Treatment Conservative treatment may effect a temporary cure but surgical intervention is usually required. A wide variety of surgical procedures are used with variable results and it is recognized that simple nail avulsion leads to an unacceptably high recurrence rate. Wedge resection of the nail followed by ablation of the germinal matrix with liquified phenol is a simple and effective cure with a low recurrence rate.

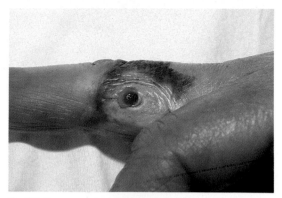

Fig. 142 Recurrence of pyogenic granuloma treated with silver nitrate.

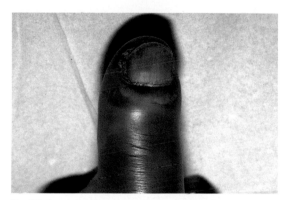

Fig. 143 A paronychia.

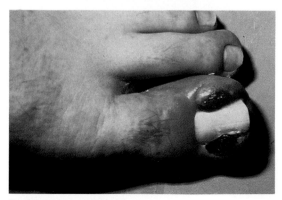

Fig. 144 An ingrowing toe nail.

Unusual conditions

Erysipelas

Erysipelas (Fig. 145) is a streptococcal infection of skin and subcutaneous tissue.

Clinical features — The lesion is sharply demarcated and has a palpable edge. The face is most commonly affected and there may be associated systemic upset requiring hospital admission.

Treatment — Treatment is with oral or intramuscular penicillin.

Orf

Orf (Fig. 146) is an infection of the skin of viral aetiology. It occurs commonly on the hands of those working with sheep.

Clinical features — It presents with a localized, painless maculopapular rash which vesiculates. This may then break down, become painful and secondarily infected.

Treatment — Treatment is with topical idoxuridine with appropriate systemic antibiotics if secondary infection has developed. It should not be drained surgically despite its appearance.

Anthrax

Anthrax (Fig. 147) is a now rare bacterial infection which also occurs predominantly in farmers and in those workers who handle animal skins.

Clinical features — It produces a pruritic red papule which vesiculates and progresses to a painless black eschar with marked surrounding non-pitting oedema. There may be systemic upset.

Treatment — Treatment is with regular intramuscular penicillin.

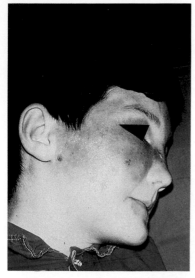

Fig. 145 Erysipelas requiring hospitalization.

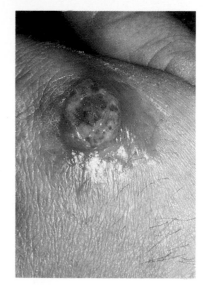

Fig. 146 Orf.

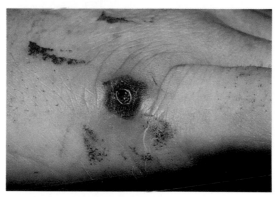

Fig. 147 The black eschar of anthrax.

24 / Burns

Aetiology   These are due to corrosive chemicals, heat, electricity or some other high energy source. The damage to the skin and deeper tissues depends upon the duration of contact and the temperature or energies involved.

Scalds

Scalds occur from hot liquid or steam, and are usually superficial. They are moist, red, blistered and exquisitely painful as the nerve endings are intact (Fig. 148).

Treatment   These are treated conservatively by dressing with non-adherent dressings and they heal spontaneously within 14 days. Extensive blisters (Fig. 149) should not be deroofed as this leaves a very sensitive area—just aspirate and dress.

Deep burns

The full extent may take some days to become apparent. They develop slough on the burned area and the sensation is impaired. Full-thickness burns are charred (Fig. 150), the skin is anaesthetic due to destruction of nerve endings and feels firm. Coagulated blood in the subcutaneous vessels shows through the burned skin.

Treatment   Surgical débridement followed by skin grafting is required.

Inhalation injury

Facial burns are usually superficial and, because of the good blood supply, heal very quickly. They are treated by exposure rather than by dressing. Alarming swelling may develop within the first 48 hours and this can impair the airway, particularly if there has been inhalation of smoke or other hot gas (Fig. 151). Look for singeing of nasal hair and the presence of intra-oral soot. If in doubt, contact an anaesthetist with a view to early intubation to protect the airway.

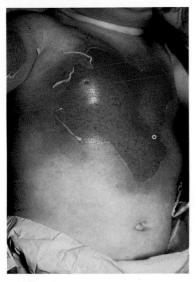

Fig. 148 A scald from hot water.

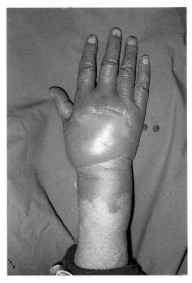

Fig. 149 A large blister on a hand.

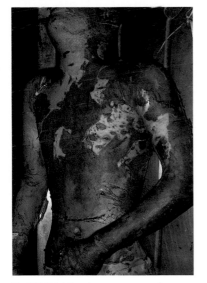

Fig. 150 Fatal deep burns.

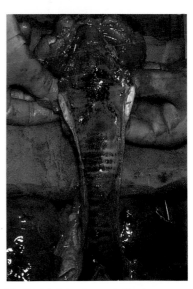

Fig. 151 Inhalation damage to the airway.

Chemical burns

These usually occur in accidents in laboratories or industrial plants but may occasionally be self-inflicted (Fig. 152). They often involve acids or alkalis but may also involve a variety of organic chemicals.

Treatment   Treatment is by washing the area liberally with running water. Some specific antidotes exist, such as topical calcium gluconate gel or calcium gluconate injection locally for hydrofluoric acid, and topical sodium bicarbonate solution for acid burns. Burns with alkali are more serious than with acid because the alkali penetrates the skin and continues to burn the subcutaneous tissue, resulting in a deeper burn than is first anticipated. A little-appreciated problem is that cement is alkaline and may cause extensive burns of the legs and feet (Fig. 153) if spillage over the top of boots is not recognized and treated immediately.

Hand burns

These usually result in marked swelling.

Treatment   Superficial burns are treated conservatively by elevation and application of silver sulphadiazine cream, followed by enclosing the hand in a loosely fitting plastic bag. This is to minimize swelling and encourage active mobilization of the fingers from the earliest possible time. This can result in a rather alarming appearance (Fig. 154) which needs to be explained to the patient.

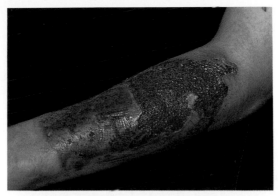

Fig. 152 Self-inflicted burns with acid to destroy a tattoo.

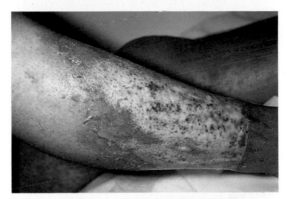

Fig. 153 'Wellington boot' cement burn. Note the line of the sock.

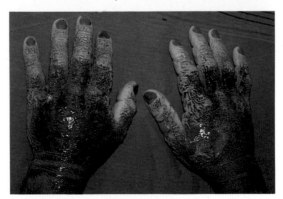

Fig. 154 Burn of the hand treated with a large glove and silver sulphadiazine.

25 / **Wound care**

General Wounds may be incised, that is made with a sharp object, or be lacerated, that is have irregular edges and be made by a blunt object or by tearing the skin. Always elicit an accurate history of the aetiology so as to be aware of possible complications or forensic connotations. Beware of a stab wound as the size of the skin wound bears little relation to the depth and direction of the wound track.

Closure Most wounds can be closed by suture. Adhesive tapes (Fig. 155) can be used in superficial wounds and obviate the need for local anaesthesia. This is of particular value in children. Histoacryl skin cement is used occasionally, particularly to close scalp wounds.

Problems Wounds more than 8 hours old are likely to be contaminated. They should be cleaned thoroughly, left open and considered for secondary suture after a period of 3 or 4 days. This reduces the risk of infection and subsequent wound breakdown.

A knuckle wound (Fig. 156) which has resulted from a blow to a victim's mouth may have produced tendon and joint capsular injuries. These are not obvious if the finger is examined with the finger extended. They require antibiotic cover and careful review.

If a wound looks as if it needs another suture, it probably does. If it looks as if it has been sutured too tightly, it has and will result in tissue necrosis (Fig. 157).

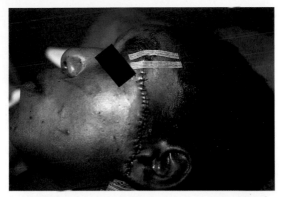

Fig. 155 Facial sutures and adhesive tapes.

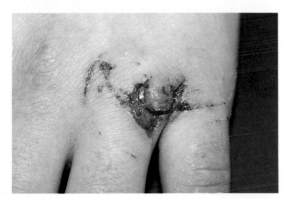

Fig. 156 A 4-day-old punch wound is best left open.

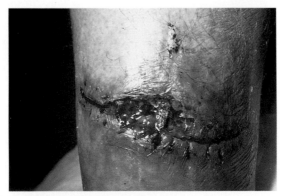

Fig. 157 Wound breakdown produced by suturing too tightly.

Exploration All wounds must be explored thoroughly under local or
general anaesthetic. If bleeding cannot be controlled by
direct pressure, a tourniquet can be applied for a short
period. When exploring a wound, first exclude the
presence of foreign material. If some is found, check that
there is no more. Consider carefully each structure in the
area of the wound and check its integrity, even if clinical
examination shows apparently full function of
neurovascular and tendinous structures. Nerve injuries
in the hand or proximal parts of the fingers warrant
careful surgical repair.

Cut tendons can be missed easily (Figs 158 & 159).
Initially there may be a partial division which may
progress subsequently to a complete rupture, particularly
when the initial discomfort has subsided and the patient
uses the limb normally. Alternatively, when examined
clinically, the patient may be in too much pain to move
the limb properly and so a divided tendon may be
suspected when this is not the case.

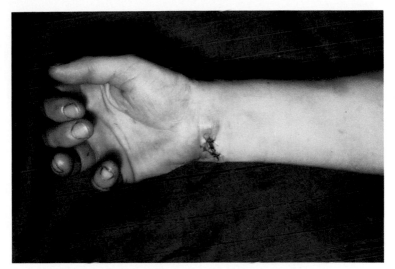

Fig. 158 Cut flexor tendon to the ring finger.

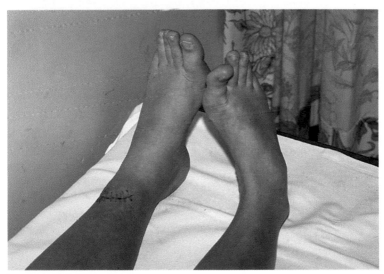

Fig. 159 Cut tibialis anterior tendon from glass.

Pretibial wounds

Clinical features   These do not heal very well in any age group but healing is particularly slow in postmenopausal women. The subcutaneous tissue is thin and the skin is friable. There is often a flap of tissue which rolls back like a roller blind and so the surface epithelium is in contact with the subcutaneous tissue and does not heal (Fig. 160).

Treatment   The flap should be cleaned thoroughly and replaced gently to its normal position. It may be held in place using absorbable subcutaneous sutures sparingly or the use of steristrips. More recently, Histoacryl glue has been used to anchor the fragile skin edges with success. The skin should not be sutured as this results in necrosis of the flap (Fig. 161). Alternatively, the flap may be 'de-fatted' and used as a fenestrated in-situ graft, being held with a few, lightly tied sutures (Figs 162 & 163). This gives valuable cover to a potentially extensive wound. The patient must rest with the leg elevated but active mobilization around the house is advised towards the end of the first week.

The wound is dressed with a non-adherent dressing such as tulle-gras or Viscopaste. The wound may break down to form an ulcer which requires dressings until healing has occurred and this may take 12 weeks.

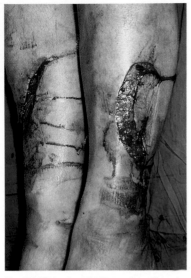

Fig. 160 Bilateral pretibial lacerations. Note the roller blind edge on the left leg.

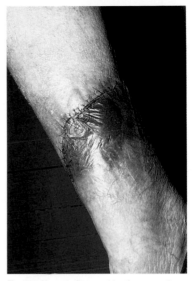

Fig. 161 Necrotic flap resulting from suturing.

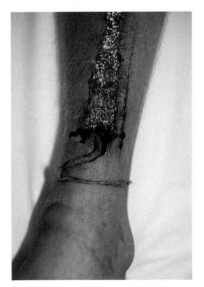

Fig. 162 Large pretibial wound with the base of the flap intact.

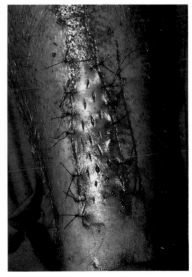

Fig. 163 A fenestrated in-situ graft using the flap.

Pretibial haematoma

This is very painful due to the tense swelling. There is a tendency for the skin over the haematoma to necrose because of the pressure (Fig. 164).

Treatment Ideally, the haematoma should be drained before necrosis occurs. Aspiration is associated with recurrence so the skin should be incised and a surprisingly large volume of coagulated blood will be evacuated. If skin necrosis has occurred, this must be removed (Fig 165). The wound should be packed lightly with non-adherent material and a firm dressing applied. Further treatment is as for a pretibial laceration.

Dog bites

Treatment The wound should be cleaned thoroughly, and wounds on the face (Fig. 166) may be closed carefully to produce a good cosmetic result. Extensive wounds elsewhere may also be closed, but it is important that suturing should be done lightly to allow escape of any exudate which may collect. Small wounds are cleaned thoroughly and left open. Do not forget to check the tetanus immunity of the patient and consider antibiotics, particularly if the wound is old or signs of infection are present at first consultation.

Fish hooks

Treatment Under local anaesthetic, push the barb through the skin in the same direction as its entry (Fig. 167). Cut the hook with wire cutters and remove it.

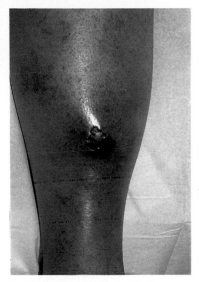

Fig. 164 Pretibial haematoma with skin necrosis.

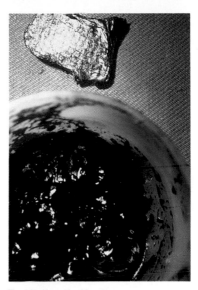

Fig. 165 Necrotic skin with evacuated haematoma.

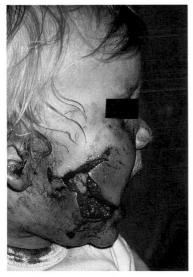

Fig. 166 Dog bite to the face.

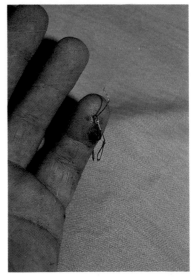

Fig. 167 Fish hook in the finger.

26 / **Foreign bodies**

Aetiology Foreign bodies in the limbs are usually due to injuries from glass or falling on to fragmented material. Wooden foreign bodies occur less commonly and are usually due to gardening accidents. Foreign bodies in the head, neck or trunk are likely to result from a missile (Fig. 168) or an assault.

Clinical features It is important to examine neurovascular and tendinous function of a limb distal to the wound. Glass and metal are radio-opaque and an X-ray is mandatory. A wooden foreign body will not necessarily show on X-ray unless there is any associated paint on the wood or air outlines the fragment.

Localization of the foreign body by radiography involves two X-rays at right angles (Fig. 169). Metallic skin markers should be used since they give a guide to the direction and depth of the foreign material in relation to the markers whose outline should be drawn on the skin over the entry wound (Fig. 170).

Treatment Foreign bodies are notoriously difficult to remove, even under ideal operating conditions which include general anaesthesia, a bloodless field and an operating theatre.

Foreign bodies in the chest or abdomen must be suspected of having damaged deeper structures. Intravenous access must be established and resuscitation undertaken as appropriate before referral to a surgeon for formal exploration.

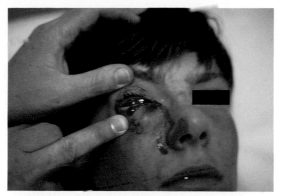

Fig. 168 Air gun pellet wound to the right eye.

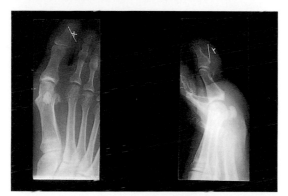

Fig. 169 Anteroposterior and lateral films of a needle in the great toe.

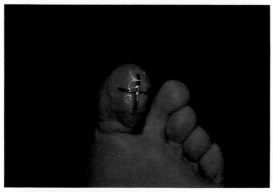

Fig. 170 Pieces of paper clip used as skin markers.

27 / **Plastering**

If appropriately trained plaster room staff are not available 24 hours a day, A & E staff should familiarize themselves with the basic techniques to stabilize a fracture until a definitive cast can be applied. The aims are to prevent displacement at the fracture site and to preserve both the blood and nerve supplies to the limb.

Materials   Several casting materials are available. Traditionally, calcium sulphate (plaster of Paris) impregnated bandages are used and these are easy to apply either in bandage or plaster slab form.

Resin materials are lighter and more comfortable for the patient but demand much more experience to apply correctly.

Common casts   A & E staff should be competent in the application of common casts such as a back slab (Fig. 171), a scaphoid (Fig. 172) and a below knee cast (Fig. 173). It is more comfortable for the patient to have an injured limb immobilized with a cast or back slab than to use a bulky 'wool and crêpe' bandage which is likely to slip.

Technique   A layer of protective material is applied to the limb prior to the casting material to protect the underlying skin. In general, the fracture site is immobilized as well as the joints above and below the site of injury. The limb is immobilized in a position of function whenever possible but there are notable exceptions such as a Smith's fracture which is immobilized with the wrist in full dorsiflexion.

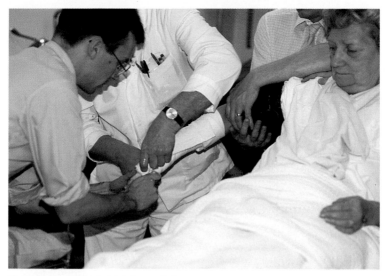

Fig. 171 A forearm back slab being applied.

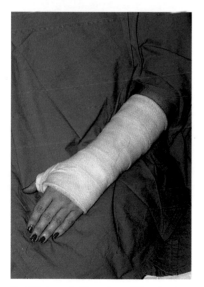

Fig. 172 A scaphoid cast immobilizes the thumb.

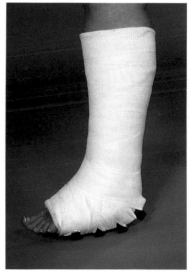

Fig. 173 A below-knee resin cast with a walking heel.

Complications

Swelling During the early period following an injury, there may
be little bruising and swelling. This increases over the
first 72 hours so any cast should be well padded to allow
for this swelling. A patient who returns complaining of
any swelling (Fig. 174), and has clinical evidence of
neurovascular compression, must have the cast split
longitudinally or removed (Fig. 175). If split, it must be
split down to skin since the padding material beneath
the cast may also compromise the circulation.

Pressure sores Moulding the cast by pressing the fingers on the wet cast
will cause friction between the cast and skin and may
result in blister formation which will break down and
may become infected or necrose. A patient must be
discouraged from inserting anything between the cast
and skin (Fig. 176) because this also can lead to a
pressure sore.

If a patient complains of increased pain at the site of
an injury beneath the cast, a window should be cut in the
cast to allow the underlying skin to be inspected. If the
skin has not broken down, the cast can be restored and a
further layer of cast material used to hold the window in
place. If there is evidence of skin ischaemia or necrosis,
specific treatment can be given and the window replaced
temporarily, allowing daily inspection of the skin.

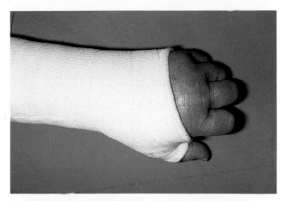

Fig. 174 Swelling of the hand distal to a scaphoid cast.

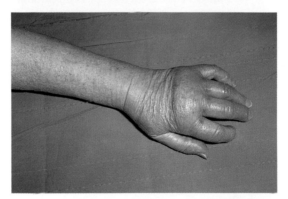

Fig. 175 The same hand (Fig. 174) after removal of the cast.

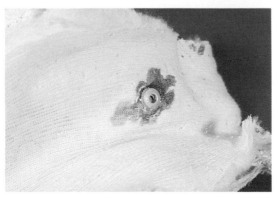

Fig. 176 Source of irritation and skin necrosis—the end off a knitting needle!

28 / Gunshot wounds and blast injuries

Gunshot wounds

Features   Gunshot wounds are divided into high velocity from rifles and low velocity from hand guns. High velocity wounds are most common in a war or terrorist situation. They are associated with massive tissue damage and are characterized by a small entry and a large exit wound. Low velocity wounds are associated with damage confined to structures in the bullet's path (Fig. 177). The bullet may follow tissue planes and remain in the patient at some distance from its expected position. Check that the number of wounds correlates with the number of bullets seen on X-ray (Fig. 178).

Treatment   This depends upon the nature and position of the wound. Try to determine the entry and exit points and the possible course followed by the bullet. Resuscitation and surgical exploration are indicated.

Bomb blasts

Features   The injuries produced depend upon the size of the explosion, whether it was in an enclosed space and the distance between it and the patient. Injuries result from the blast wave and flash as well as fragments of masonry or metal energized by the blast (Fig. 179).

Treatment   Careful assessment, resuscitation and awareness of possible pressure damage to the ear and lung.

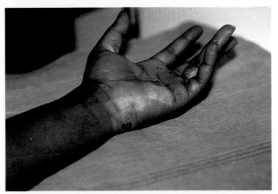

Fig. 177 Entry and exit wounds in a hand holding a bottle.

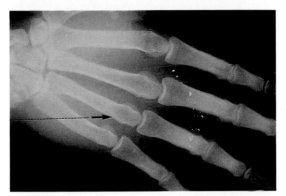

Fig. 178 Line of bullet. The foreign bodies are glass, and not bullet fragments.

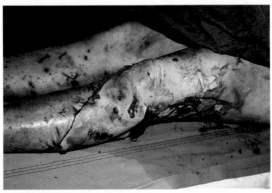

Fig. 179 Flash and shrapnel wounds from a bomb explosion.

Diagnosis   The greatest care must be taken to neither miss nor misdiagnose these injuries. It takes time and experience to differentiate an accidental from a non-accidental injury (Fig. 180) so senior colleagues, who have specific experience in this field, should be consulted.

Clinical features   Factors which may alert the attending doctor to the problem include:

- the patient is already identified on the 'at risk' register
- the patient might be a frequent attender at the A & E department
- the parents or guardians give a variable history which does not fit the clinical signs (Fig. 181)
- there may be an unusual distribution of injury with an unusual appearance, such as bruising well away from bony prominences (Fig. 182)
- there may be radiological evidence of old, multiple bony injuries
- the child has a wary, worried expression and does not interact normally with other children or experienced staff on the ward.

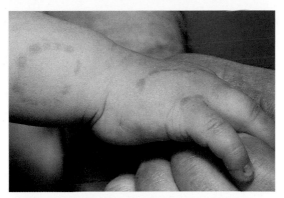

Fig. 180 Human bite marks on the distal forearm and hand.

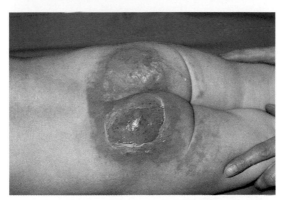

Fig. 181 'Bath dipping'—typically the scalds are on the buttocks and feet.

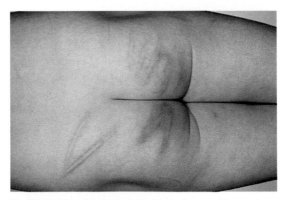

Fig. 182 Bruising of the buttocks from being beaten with a wooden stick.

30 / Miscellaneous problems

Self-inflicted wounds

Repeated superficial lacerations on accessible parts of the body (Fig. 183) are often more a cry for help than an attempt at suicide. The wound may require surgical treatment but consider the whole patient as the wound is only a small part of the problem. The patient's psychological state must be assessed and, if indicated, the help of a psychiatrist should be enlisted. Follow-up must be arranged via the general practitioner if the patient is registered but avoid situations where there may be a long delay in such follow-up.

Delivery in A & E

Occasionally a mother will give sudden and unexpected birth whilst in the department (Fig. 184). The mother is usually young, single and will have concealed the fact that she is pregnant. She will not have had any antenatal care. Share in the joy of a healthy delivery and ensure that there is both social and obstetric follow-up.

Iatrogenic problems

Treatment sometimes causes problems. One of the most common is a reaction to a tetanus toxoid injection (Fig. 185). This produces swelling and erythema as well as local pain. The patient should be reassured, treated symptomatically and followed up until the problem has settled.

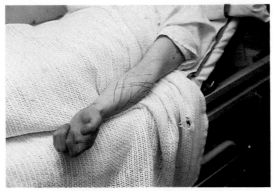
Fig. 183 Self-inflicted lacerations to the wrist and forearm.

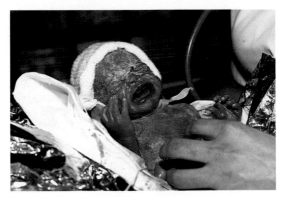
Fig. 184 Delivery in the A & E department.

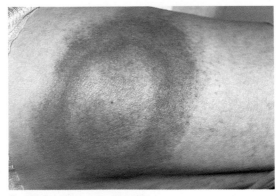
Fig. 185 Reaction to tetanus toxoid.

31 / **Dangers to staff**

Protect yourself It is essential that members of staff always take precautions against contamination from patients' body fluids. Patients seen in an A & E department are mostly unknown to staff and, in situations such as major trauma or unconsciousness from alcohol or drugs, no history will be available. Assume that all patients are an infection hazard and make sure to wear gloves as the minimum protection (Fig. 186) whenever you are carrying out any invasive procedure such as venepuncture, cannulation or endotracheal intubation. Gloves must also be worn when dealing with an open wound.

High risk If there is a case of a known HIV or hepatitis positive patient (Fig. 187), senior medical staff should be involved and full protective measures taken as appropriate, which may include the use of gowns, an apron, mask, visor and double gloves.

Low risk Do not forget the less melodramatic infection hazards of an A & E department such as fleas, lice and scabies (Fig. 188). They are still very common, particularly in homeless individuals. Medical and nursing staff probably remain the greatest hazard to themselves and to other members of the hospital staff due to carelessness. Ensure that you personally dispose of all needles and sharps in a safe manner.

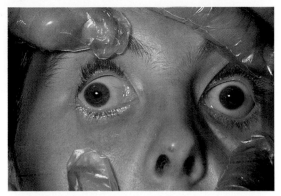

Fig. 186 A patient with Hepatitis B—note that the doctor is wearing gloves.

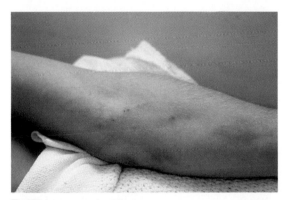

Fig. 187 Intravenous drug abuse.

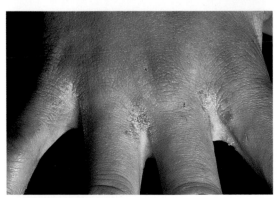

Fig. 188 Common site of burrows in scabies.

Index

Abscess, 105, 106
  ischiorectal/perianal, 69, 70
Achilles tendon, rupture, 95, 96
Acromioclavicular injury, 41, 42
Airway
  foreign bodies, 21, 22, 27, 28
  hot gas/smoke inhalation damaging, 111, 112
Allergy, skin, 101, 102
Amputation, fingertip, 61–2
Anal area/region, conditions affecting, 67–72
Ankle, 93–6
Anthrax, 109, 110
Arm, 43–4, *see also* Elbow; Hand; Wrist

Biceps muscle, damage, 43–4
Biceps tendinitis, 47–8
Bier's block, 49, 50
Birth in A & E, 133, 134
Bite, dog, 121, 122
Blast injury, 129–30
Bleeding/haemorrhage, *see also* Haematoma
  from ear, 13, 14
  into eye (anterior chamber), 15, 16
  nasal, 23, 24
  tooth socket, 21, 22
  from varicose veins, 91
Blood, *see* Bleeding; Haematoma
Bomb blasts, 129, 130
Bones, ankle, conditions affecting, 95
Boutonnière deformity, 57, 58
Burns, 111–14
Bursitis, 97–8
  calcific, 41, 42

Cancer, skin, 103, 104
Cannulation, central venous, 9, 10
Carcinoma, squamous cell, 103, 104
Cardiac massage, 7
Cardiac tamponade, 9, 10
Casts, plaster, 125–8
Catheters/catheterization
  central venous, 9, 10
  contraindications and complications, 75, 77, 78
Cellulitis, 105, 106
Central venous cannulation, 9, 10
Cervical collar, 33, 34
Cervical spine, sprain, 33
Chemical burns, 113, 114
Chest pain, traumatic, 37–8
Collateral ligaments of knee, injury, 85, 86
Colles fracture, 49, 50
Compartment syndrome, 91, 92
Conjunctivitis, 17, 18
Corneal foreign bodies, 17, 18
Cranial (skull) fractures, 12, 13–14
Cutaneous conditions, 99–104

Cyst, infected, 105, 106

Dangers to staff, 135–6
Defibrillation, 6, 7, 8
Degloving injury, 65, 66
Delivery in A & E, 133, 134
Dendritic ulcer, 19, 20
Dental problems, 21–2
Dermal conditions, 99–104
Digits, *see* Fingers; Toes
Dislocation
  ankle, 95, 96
  hip, 79, 80
  jaw, 25, 26
  lunate, 51
  nail/nail root, 59, 60
  patellar, 87, 88
  shoulder, 39, 40
Dog bite, 121, 122

Ear, 29–32
  bleeding from 13, 14
  pain, 29–32
Eczema, 101, 102
Elbow, 45–8
Epicondylar epiphysis, medial, separation, 45, 46
Epicondylitis, 47, 48
Epiphysis, epicondylar, medial, separation, 45, 46
Episcleritis, 17
Epistaxis, 23, 24
Erysipelas, 109, 110
Eye conditions, 15–20

Femoral neck fracture, 79, 80
Femoral nerve block, 81, 82
Femoral vessels, damage, 81, 82
Finger injury, 57–8, 61–2, 65, 66, 118, *see also* Kunckle; Nail
Fish hooks, 121, 122
Fissure in-ano (anal fissure), 67
Flexor tendon/tendon sheath
  cut, 118
  infection, 63
Foreign bodies, 123–4
  airway, 21, 22, 27, 28
  ear, 31, 32
  eye, 17, 18
  rectum, 71–2
  throat, 27, 28
Fractures
  femoral neck, 79, 80
  hand/finger, 65, 66
  jaw, 25
  malleolus (lateral), 95, 96
  orbital, 15, 16

pelvic, 75
scaphoid, 55–6
skull, 12, 13–14
wrist, 49, 50, 51, 52

Gastrocnemius muscle pain, 91, 92
Gentiourinary problems, 73–8
Glaucoma, 19
Gonorrhoea, 73, 74
Grafts
  for amputated fingertip, 61, 62
  fenestrated in-situ, 119, 120
Granuloma, pyogenic, 107, 108
Groin, 81–2
Gun wounds, 36, 123, 129–30

Haemarthrosis in knee, 83, 84
Haematoma
  nasal septa, 23, 24
  perianal, 67
  perichondral (ear), 31, 32
  perineal, 75
  pretibial, 121, 122
  subungual, 59
Haemorrhage, see Bleeding
Haemorrhoids, 67, 68
Hand, 57–66, see also Finger; Knuckle; Wrist
  burns, 113, 114
  swollen, 49
Hazards to staff, 135–6
Head injury, 11–14
Hepatitis infection, staff, 135
Herpes simplex infection, 99
  genital, 73, 74
Herpes zoster infection, 99, 100
High pressure injection injury of finger, 65, 66
Hip pain, 79–80
HIV infection, staff, 135
Hyphaema, 15, 16

Iatrogenic problems, 133, 134
Infection
  ear, 29
  genital, 73, 74
  hand, 63–4
  hazards to staff, 135
  perianal, 67, 69–70
  skin, 99–100
  soft tissue, 105–10
Inflammation, see also Pain
  bursal sac, see Bursitis
  conjunctival, 17, 18
  ear, 29–30
  epicondylar, 47, 48
  iris, 19, 20
  scleral/episcleral, 17
  tendon, see Biceps tendinitis;
    Tenosynovitis
  urethral, gonococcal, 73, 74

vulvovaginal, herpetic, 74
Inhalation
  hot gas/smoke, 111, 112
  tooth, 21, 22
Injection, high pressure, finger injury caused
    by, 65, 66
Injury, traumatic, see specific site and types of
    injury, e.g. Fracture
Iris
  inflammation (iritis), 19, 20
  prolapse, 19, 20

Jaw injury, 25, 26
Joints, ankle, conditions affecting, 95, see also
    specific joints

Keratoacanthoma, 103, 104
Knee, 83–90
Knuckle (punch) wound, 115, 116

Lateral ligaments of ankle, injury, 93, 94
Leg, 91–2, see also Ankle; Knee
Lichen planus, 101, 102
Ligament injuries
  ankle, 93–4
  knee, 85–6
Lip injury, 25, 26
Lipohaemarthrosis in knee, 83, 84
Lunate dislocation, 51
Lung, see Airway

Malignancies, skin, 103, 104
Mallet finger, 57
Mandibular injury, 25
Median nerve compression, 49, 50
Melanoma, 103, 104
Missile wounds, 36, 123, 124, 129–30
Molluscum contagiosum, 99, 100
Muscle, see specific muscle

Nail(s)
  finger
    injury, 59–60
    melanoma under, 103, 104
  toe, ingrowing, 107, 108
Nail fold, infection, 107, 108
Nasal problems, 23–4
Neck, 33–6, see also Throat
Non-accidental injury, 131–2
Nose problem, 23–4

Ocular problems, 15–20
Olecranon bursa, 98
Ophthalmological problems, 15–20
Orbital fractures, 15, 16
Orf, 109, 110
Orofacial conditions, 21–8
Otitis externa, 29, 30
Otitis media, 29

Pain, see also inflammation
  chest, 37–8
  ear, 29–32

eye, 17–20
hip, 79–80
knee, 87–8
leg muscle, 91
neck, 33–4
shoulder, in abduction, 41, 42
Paraphimosis, 73, 74
Paronychia, 107, 108
Patellar dislocation, 87, 88
Pelvic fractures, 75
Penetrating injuries, *see* Perforating injuries
Perforating/penetrating injuries
chest, 37, 38
eye, 19, 20
Perianal conditions, 67–72
Perineal bruising/haematoma, 75
Physical abuse, 131–2
Pilonidal sinus/abscess, 69, 70
Pityriasis rosea, 101, 102
Plastering, 125–8
Pneumothorax, tension, 9, 10
Pressure sores, cast-associated, 127, 128
Pretibial haematoma, 121, 122
Pretibial wounds, 119–20
Punch (knuckle) wound, 115, 116
Pyogenic granuloma, 107, 108
Pyogenic infection, 105, 106
hand, 63, 64

Quadriceps
ruptured, 87, 88
wasting, 89, 90

Relatives, unsuccessful resuscitation and, 5–7
Resuscitation, 5–10
Rib fracture, 37, 38
Ring finger injuries, 65, 66, 118
Rodent ulcer, 103, 104

Safety practices, 135–6
Scabies infection, staff, 135
Scalds, 111, 112, 132
Scalp wounds, 11, 12
Scaphoid, fractured, 55–6
Scleritis, 17
Self-inflicted injury, 133, 134
burns, 113, 114
neck/throat, 35, 36
Shoulder, 39–42
Skin conditions, 99–104
Skull fractures, 12, 13–14
Smith's fracture, 51, 52
Soft tissues
infection, 105–10
wrist, conditions affecting, 53–4
Spine, cervical, *see entries under* Cervical
Sprain, cervical spine, 33
Squamous tell carcinoma, 103, 104
Staff, 1–3
dangers to, 135–6
Subungual haematoma, 59, 60

Subungual melanoma, 103, 104
Swelling
casts causing, 127, 128
hand, 49
over tendons in wrist, 53, 54
Synovial irritation, 83
Synovitis, bursal, *see* Bursitis

Team, *see* Staff
Teeth, problems with, 21–2
Tendinitis, biceps, 47–8
Tendon(s)
Achilles, rupture, 95, 96
cut, 117, 118
in hand
infection, 63
injury, 57–8, 118
inflammation, *see* Tendinitis;
Tenosynovitis
in wrist, swelling over, 53, 54
Tenosynovitis, 53
Testicular torsion, 77, 78
Tetanus toxoid reaction, 133, 134
Threadworm infection, 67
Throat problems, 27–8, *see also* Neck
Tibialis anterior tendon, cut, 118
Tinel's sign, 49, 50
Toe nail, ingrowing, 107, 108
Tooth problems, 21–2
Torticollis, 33, 34
Trauma, *see specific site*
Tumours, skin, 103–4

Ulcer
dendritic, 19, 20
varicose, 91
Ungual problems, *see entries under* Nail;
Subungual
Urethra
inflammation (urethritis), gonococcal, 7⟨
trauma, 75, 76
Urine retention, 77, 78

Varicose veins, 91, 92
Veins
central, cannulation, 9, 10
varicose, 91, 92
Ventricular fibrillation, 7
Virus infections of skin, 99–100
Volar plate deformity, 57
Vulvovaginitis, herpetic, 74

Warts, 99, 100
Wounds
care, 115–22
types and sites, *see specific types/sites*
Wrist, 49–56, *see also* Hand